I0447631

Point of View

POV on Dying and Living
How My Life-Threatening Tumor Redefined Me

DEBBIE BERKELHAMMER

ISBN: 1477453709

ISBN 13: 9781477453704

CreateSpace title ID#: 3875811

Library of Congress Control Number: 2012915943

CreateSpace Independent Publishing Platform

North Charleston, South Carolina

~Dedicated to my sons, Josh and Alex~

~Written in honor of the story that lives within us all~

Preface

In the final hours of darkness, just before the sun would break and the next day's cocktail was consumed, I would lie still in my bed, feeling most like myself. It was in these moments I faced my greatest fears in true consciousness. The buzzing was gone from my brain and my mind clear to wander through the darkness that had descended on my family and me. I was thirty-one years old and had been given one to three months to live. A morning cocktail of steroids and Xanax would weave its way through my body, into my blood; the steroids were an upper and caused the jitters and a constant buzzing in my head; the Xanax was a downer and kept my emotions, well, nonexistent. I spent each moment of daylight buzzing and depressed. I was a shell of the woman I once knew. I would lie awake at night, whole for the moment, drug free; the thoughts of not *being* rocking me to my core. That was my truest sadness and fear, and I would cry for my sons.

I didn't fear being replaced. I feared for the empty space in their life that used to be me. After I was gone, would they close their eyes at night and feel the warmth of my lips on their foreheads? Would they remember what my embrace felt like, the way I inhaled them and held on just a bit longer? Would they in turn give hugs like that? Would they hear my voice when they needed help? Would they remember how I smelled and what my skin felt like, or would those memories fade away? That this would be their destiny was such an injustice. Why should they carry a lifetime of pity from others and sadness that their mother died when they were so young? I wondered what legacy I would leave for them. I pleaded out loud, many times screaming to a God I wasn't sure existed, "Please, please, I need more time." I wasn't nearly done raising my sons. I wasn't finished, damn it! I didn't want to be gone. My sons were so young, just three and nine years old; we were in the throes of life. I would imagine the pain that would be left for them to trudge through without me.

It wasn't just the lessons in life I was afraid of not teaching, but the moments in life I couldn't bear to miss. These were moments I was supposed to have. How dare this tumor steal *my* moments? The image of my sons' faces and the emptiness in their hearts was enough to cause me to curl into a fetal position and sob uncontrollably, or stare into space and look for ways to make this nightmare go away. The darkness brought my mind and body to an even level, but I admit the emotions were so excruciating there were mornings I savaged my meds so that I could free myself from my reality. But then night would fall on me again and reality would force its way back in.

Dear Reader,

I was thirty years old when my pediatric spinal cord tumor was discovered. Less than a year later, doctors told me I had one to three months to live. I was a thirty-one-year-old mother to my young boys, Josh and Alex, and a stepmom to Cary. I was a wife, a daughter, a younger sister, and a friend to many. Today I am forty-six. When I decided it was time to write my story, I wanted my book to be more than a history of my illness. I wanted to share my point of view—my most intimate thoughts and moments during my illness and how I have transitioned to the person I am today.

I had so many roles when the illness invaded my life and everything changed. The illness first dissected me, and then ultimately lifted me up as an individual and taught me what it took to start winning again.

History is important, so I will give you the *Cliff Notes* version of my particular illness. Experience my POV on death, then life.

At the end of each chapter, there is space for you to journal your thoughts about your own experiences or perhaps those of a loved one. It's your space to just write. My memoir becomes yours.

Life is a journey, and the road is bumpy and sometimes impossible to pass, but I was lucky enough to come out of something horrific and life-changing. I want to share my story to offer comfort, compassion, hope, acceptance, and even humor to others, and so that I can continue to embrace those things as well.

Debbie

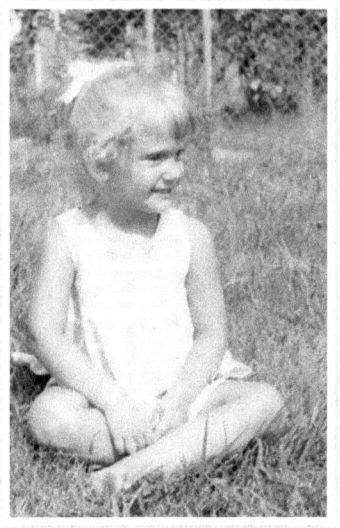

Here I am at one year old
in 1967.

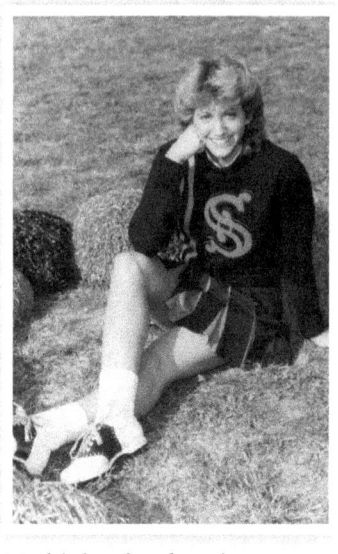

My high school senior
cheerleading picture, 1984.

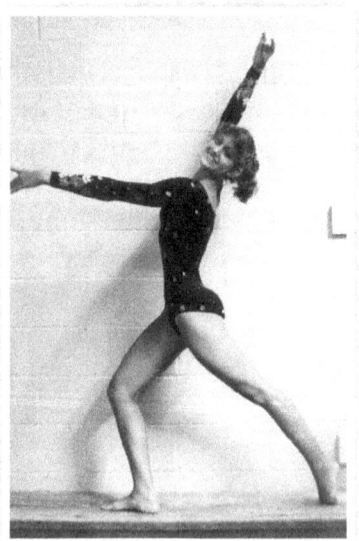

This is one of the last pictures
of me as a gymnast in 1981.

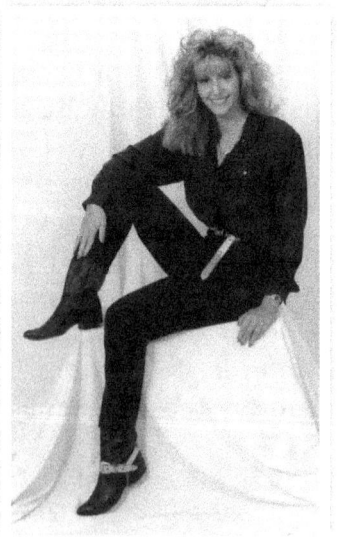

This is me in1993, three
years before I got sick.

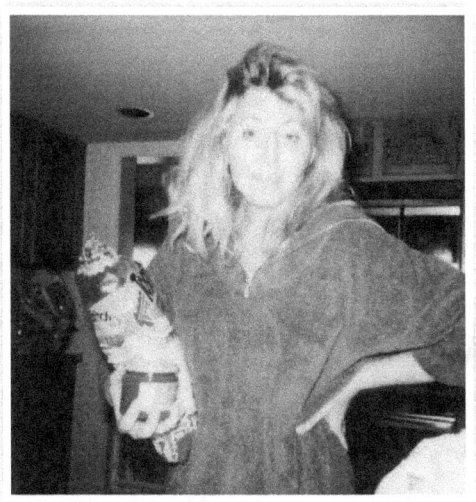

This photo was taken in October 1996,
a month after I started radiation.

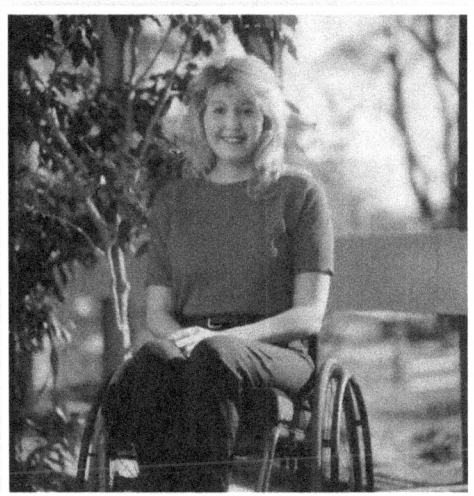

This picture was taken when I was at
Bryn Mawr Rehabilitation Hospital in
November 1996.

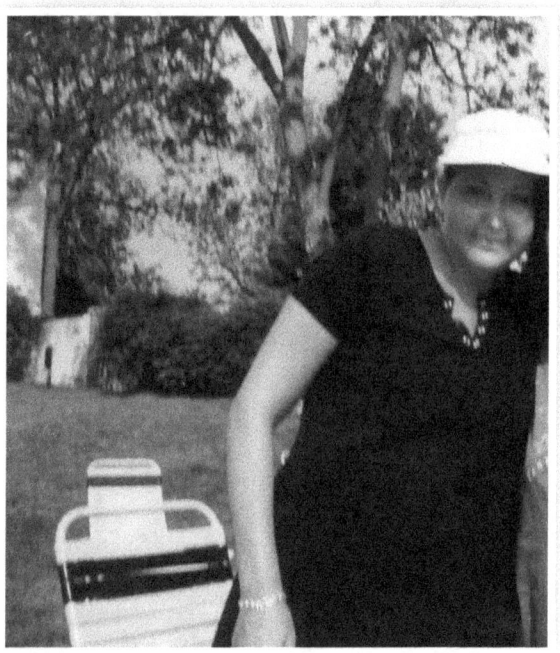

This is me in late spring 1997 after I shaved my head.

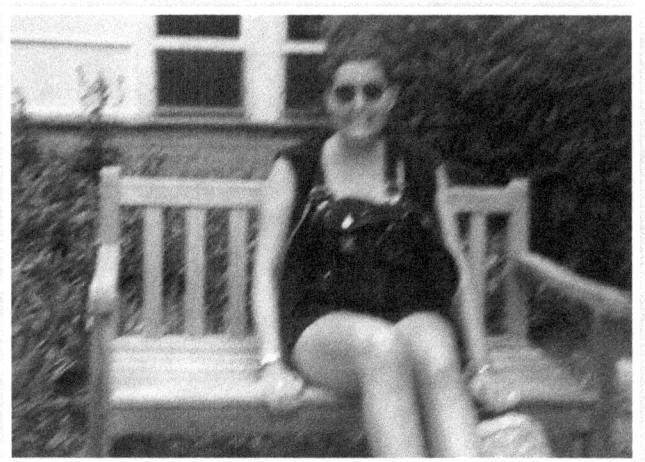

Here I am outside Alex's preschool in spring 1997.

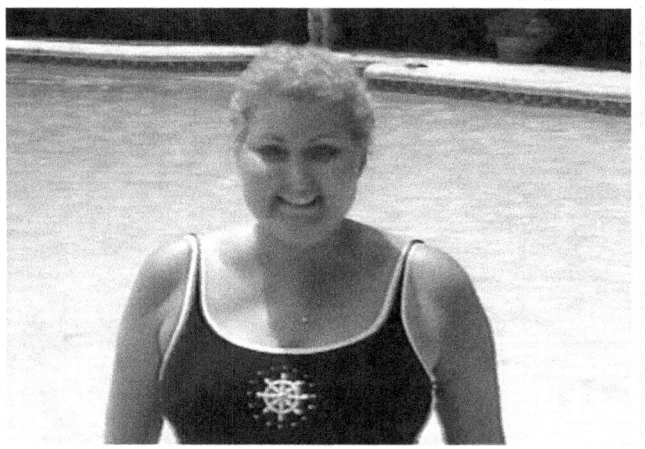

This picture was captured from the video I made June 1997, right before my second surgery.

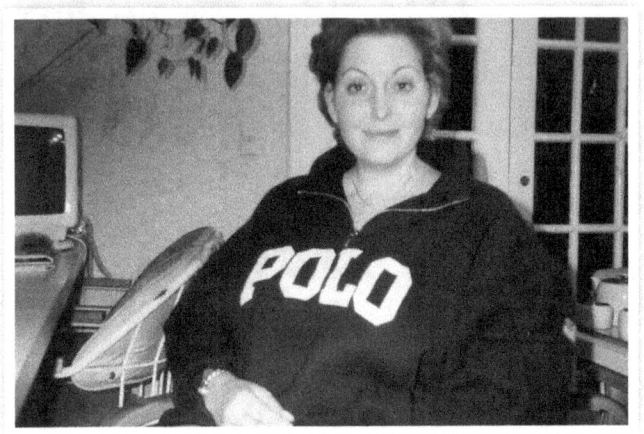

Fall 1997 after the second surgery.

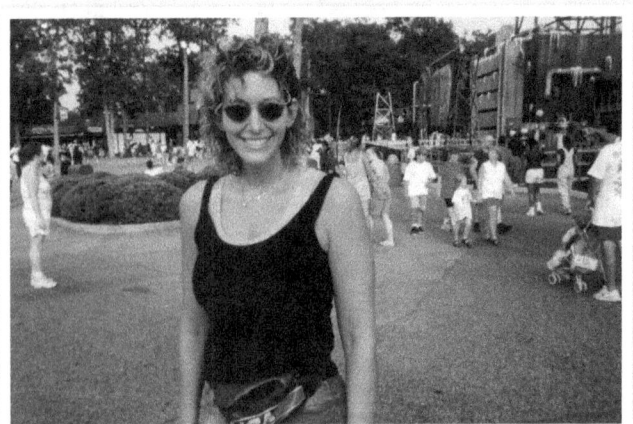

This photo was taken at an amusement park after all
surgeries were complete in spring 1998.

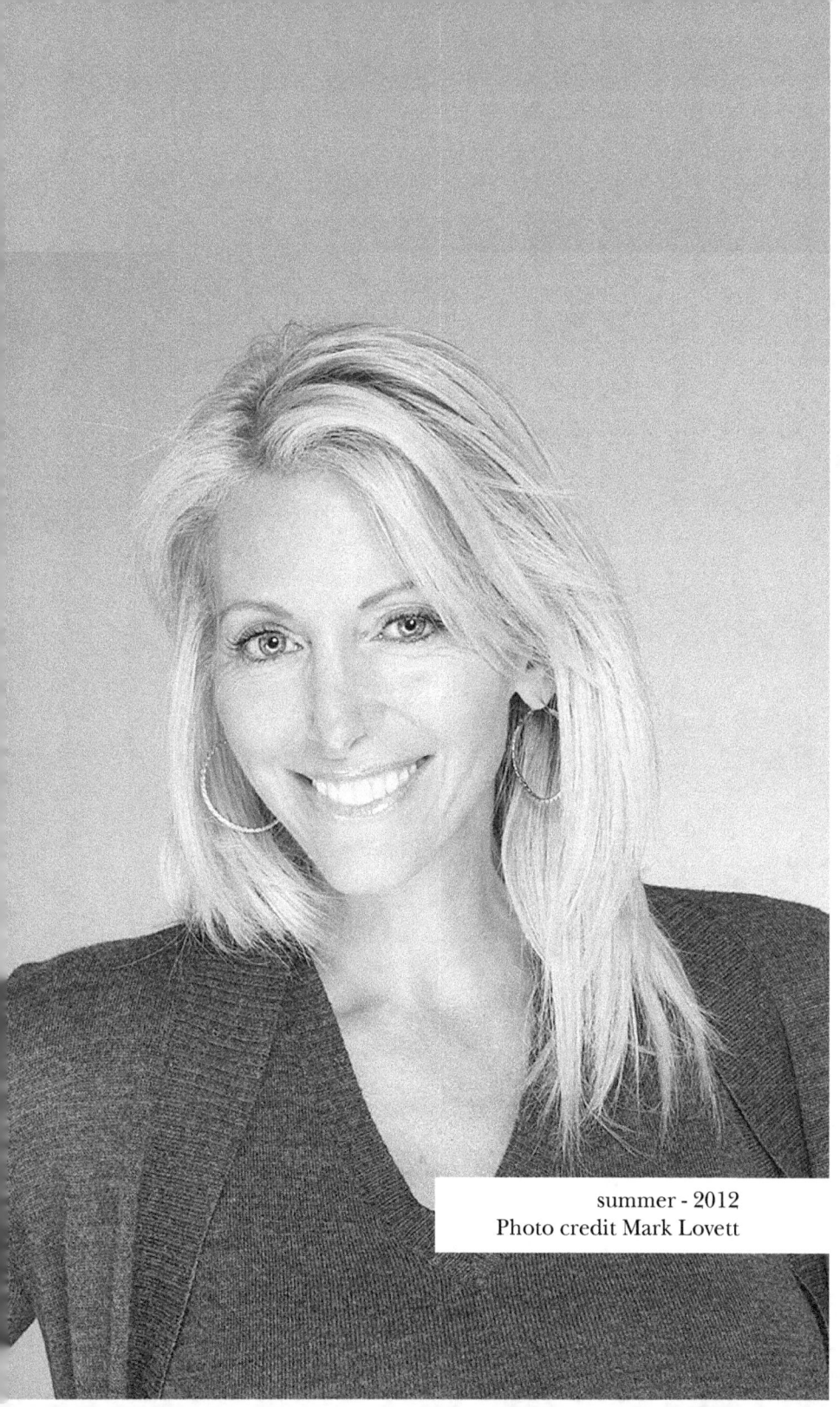

summer - 2012
Photo credit Mark Lovett

1

My Illness

In the summer of 1996, I was diagnosed with a noncancerous, life- threatening, pediatric cervical spinal-cord tumor at C2-C7. This means that my tumor had been growing inside me for most of my life. I was thirty years old; married for the second time; and the mother of two sons, Josh, from my first marriage; and Alex, from my current marriage; and a stepson, Cary. I was living in Potomac, Maryland. Up until that point, I had been an active, fit woman. In fact, most of my life had revolved around being active.

From the ages of six to sixteen, I was an advanced gymnast, training daily with Olympians and Olympic coaches. It is safe to say that being a gymnast was my life. I was shaped by my sport. Commitment, dedication, and drive were imbedded in me from an early age, pushing me to be the best in training and in competitions. Finally, after four knee surgeries, at the ripe old age of sixteen, I retired from as the activity that had been the focus of my life. As a junior in high school, I tried out for track and field, discus, and shot put. Here I was, a medium-size girl, strong as hell, and competing at state meets against girls twice my size. Then it was cheerleading. I always gave my all to everything I did. Not until later, as an adult, would I be tested again, only this time with my life.

At the time my tumor was diagnosed, I was running an advertising specialty business, where we put company logos on wearable items and novelties. and dabbling in acting and modeling. Two years prior to the discovery of the tumor, I'd had a variety of symptoms, such as shooting pains down my right arm and losing the grip in my right hand. I was dropping things. On the recommendation of my internist, I was treated for carpel tunnel syndrome and anxiety. I didn't feel I needed to see a therapist, but the doctors thought that stress might be causing my symptoms.

After almost two years, I was still seeking the reason I was not getting better. During that time, my husband, Bob, my children (then ages two and eight), and I moved to Malvern, Pennsylvania, a suburb of Philadelphia, so my husband could be closer to his son, Cary, from his previous marriage. Cary was also eight at the time.

Once in Malvern, I found an internist who took an interest in me. He ordered a magnetic resonance imaging test (MRI) of my brain and spine with a special dye, initially suspecting that I might have multiple sclerosis—MS. The process of going to get the MRI, then waiting for the results, was torturous, to say the least. Anyone who has gone through the process of diagnostic testing knows that it just plain sucks.

We got a call from my neurologist's office just a couple of days after the test; he wanted to see me the next morning. That was also a horrible moment: I knew he had found something, and no matter how much I pleaded to the nurses and even the doctor himself to please tell me the results on the phone, I had to accept that I would not know until the next day. From the minute I hung up the phone until I walked into the doctor's office the next day, everything sounded and looked different to me. I felt as though I was in slow motion; I was hoping to delay the inevitable.

The MRI confirmed that a mass was lodged in my spinal cord, pushing out my right side. Bob and I just stared at the egg-shaped, glowing thing on the films and I was silent. "How the hell did that get in there?" I asked, finally. No answers were immediately available.

Then we went into overdrive. It was a whirlwind. All of a sudden, being miles away from my family was terrifying. Someone fired the start gun; we jumped off the block, and sprinted into action. Everything around me was blurred. Getting answers was all we could think about. We called our parents, siblings, and my brother-in-law, who is a doctor. The consensus was: come back to Maryland and see a specialist. We did see a specialist in Washington, DC, and then another back in Pennsylvania. Both recommended surgery: they could not know what type of mass it was until they had removed and tested it.

I aligned myself with the best of the best doctors. The first surgeon was considered *the* workhorse in his field, the only one to go to, but when he opened me up in August 1996, he immediately closed me up. The tumor, he said, was mixed together with healthy nerve like vanilla and chocolate ice cream; if he had tried to remove it, I would have died on the operating table. His initial diagnosis was that the tumor was cancerous and inoperable. The next day, he said it was not cancer but it was inoperable and that I would be a quadriplegic at the very least in three to five years. He suggested radiation in an effort to shrink the tumor.

I went to see the head of the Neuro-Oncology and Neuro-Radiation Department at Jefferson Hospital in

Philadelphia. I then underwent six weeks of intensive radiation. I was fitted with a mask, which looked like a hockey goalie's mask, and the front of my neck was tattooed in three places. On day one and for six weeks afterward, each time I laid face up on the table in the radiation room at the hospital, the nurses would snap my mask in place and rays of radiation would enter my body. I would be remiss if I did not mention that the medication and the radiation made me horribly sick. Within weeks of starting radiation, I lost twenty pounds. I was on high levels of steroids (Decadron, to be exact), and this contributed not only to my weight loss but also to thrush, hair loss, and severe atrophy of my legs. By Thanksgiving I was a bag of bones. I had trouble walking and had to use a cane, then a walker. The week after Thanksgiving, I was rushed to the hospital by ambulance with pneumonia, a bladder infection, a high blood sugar level, and in need of a blood transfusion. I was confused, delirious, and in and out of consciousness. I spent three weeks in the hospital dealing with a new addition to my medical chart: steroid-induced diabetes. Then, because I had become so frail and unable to walk, I was sent to an inpatient physical rehabilitation center in Malvern for another two weeks.

I wish I could say that by Christmas 1996, all of this was behind me, but it wasn't.

I fired my "super" medical team when the other doctors couldn't determine which was more responsible for how sick I was—the meds or the tumor. I hired a lesser-known doctor in a smaller hospital in Paoli, Pennsylvania, and waited for test results showing that my tumor had shrunk. I continued to go to outpatient rehabilitation, but I hit rock bottom around Christmas. With my kids taking an annual trip to Florida without me, the outcome of my radiation unknown, and the person in the mirror unrecognizable, I slid deep into a depression.

I had been trying unsuccessfully to wean myself off steroids and break out of my depression. I wanted so badly to see light but I couldn't do it myself. I was so afraid I would never be able to climb back up, that I would forever be lost in this state of emptiness. Finally in late January 1997, I did it—with the help of a swift kick in the ass from my mother during my lowest, darkest point. When my mom came to stay with me during Christmas 1996, what she did for me was believe in me. She saw in me the ability to turn this darkness into light.

I gained back a few pounds and became steadier on my feet. Prozac and some much-needed positive thinking helped me get to a better place, and by the spring of 1997, I even went on a trip to Disney World with my family. (You will learn more about my mom and this encounter later in the book.) My new doctor suggested chemo, but since there was no real protocol for treating my rare tumor, I decided to just step back and take a breath, even with no evidence that the tumor had shrunk. I was buying time and trying to enjoy a moment that seemed to be free of turmoil. My hair was so thin you could see my scalp, so I shaved my head and bought a wig.

Then in June 1997, I hit a major roadblock. I had been told that paralysis was a rare side effect of radiation to the spinal cord that could show up months after treatment. I woke up just before Father's Day weekend and couldn't move. This was the day I had dreaded. I was rushed by ambulance to the hospital and put on high doses of steroids and a morphine drip.

My new doctor told me and my family that I was not experiencing a side effect of the radiation, but rather the tumor had grown. I had one to three months to live with no viable treatment option.

Bob and I and the kids moved back to Maryland to be closer to our families. I didn't pack one box; the move just happened, as if I had snapped my fingers. We moved in with my in-laws because their house had more bedrooms than my parents' home. I spent the next four weeks mostly bedridden, on morphine. Friends came by to pay their respects. The steroids then caused my weight to skyrocket; I gained sixty pounds by the time I ended up in New York for a second Hail Mary surgery in July.

Getting to New York for that surgery was nothing short of a miracle.

As I lay in bed at my in-laws', assuming death was upon me, my parents scoured the Internet for answers. I was ready to try anything. I visited holistic doctors, squeezed cotton balls, slept with marbles under my pillow, and drank green slime. Dr. Fred Epstein, a world-renowned pediatric neurosurgeon of the Institute of Neurology and Neurosurgery (INN) at Beth Israel North in New York City, turned out to be the answer. After a quick review of my diagnosis over the phone, he granted me an appointment within days. We made a side trip to Johns Hopkins Hospital, and when the very well-respected doctor I saw there said, "Well, I am not Fred Epstein," I knew I had found my man.

I was still unable to walk or sit up, so Mom and Dad and Bob loaded me on a mattress in the back of my parents' Jeep Grand Cherokee and drove me to the see the man I would come to truly believe was God.

Our meeting with Dr. Epstein was euphoric, for a lack of a better word. I swear that day I saw a glow surrounding him. Dr. Fred Epstein was the most renowned pediatric neurosurgeon in the world, and I was one of his few adult patients. The day we saw him, I was weak, engorged by steroids, and my hair was like a Brillo pad. He simply said, "I will fix you."

The list of what could happen during surgery was terrifying, but so was death. I had surgery in July 1997, staying in the hospital on the pediatric floor for four weeks.

Unfortunately, I contracted spinal meningitis while I was there, which added weeks to my recovery time. But I left in August, with 90 percent less of my tumor and a new lease on life.

I spent the next year going to outpatient physical rehabilitation in Maryland, losing weight, and getting back as much time as I could with my kids. I had to deal with the loss of most of the use of my right hand—and still do to this day; I typed this book using only my left hand.

I continue to experience severe numbness and tingling over many parts of my body, which at this point, can be attributed to side effects of the surgeries and possibly from the radiation. It took a while, but I recovered physically and emotionally. I have an MRI every two years to check on the 10 percent of the tumor that was left inside my spinal cord. There would be many changes ahead of me—in my marriage, for one; and finding a new love and losing my beloved Dr. Epstein. But I don't want to get ahead of myself.

When I talk about my illness, what resonates is how it affected my life at that time and how it still does. As I write this, it has been sixteen years since the day I went for my first set of MRIs. I have had a few scares, whiplash, and a fall on my head, and most recently increased numbness, pain, and strange vibrations throughout my body. I know there is always the possibility that the remaining 10 percent of the tumor could grow, or that another similar tumor could appear. At my lowest point, I could not summon strength and courage instantaneously. But over time, I reached deep inside to that little girl who had no fear on the balance beam and pushed forward with that same determination. I have to believe and be positive that each day will be brighter.

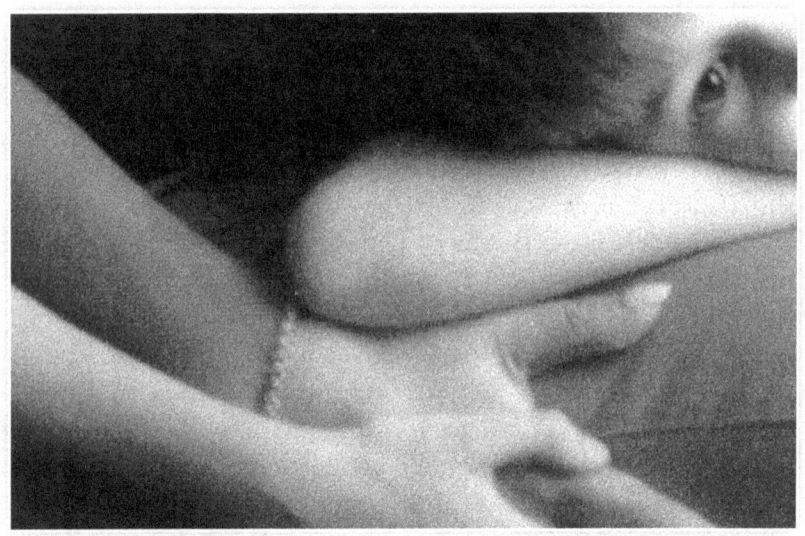

This image truly defines me. Alex's eyes, Josh's arm and mine—we are woven together, pieces of a puzzle that will always fit as one.

Photo credit: Davide Depas 2000

2

MOTHER

Definition: To give rise to or exercise protective care over something else; a person who fills those roles.

Synonyms: to tend, nurse, mind, raise

A s a mom, I was supposed to be all these things, all the time.

I have been a mom since I was twenty-one. Now my boys are men: Alex is nineteen and Josh is twenty-five. They had no choice but to go on this hideous ride with me, but I do believe it made each of us better people. Being a sick mother was *the* most difficult part of my illness. As I shared in the introduction, it wasn't the act of dying I was most afraid of—it was being gone from my sons' lives. I couldn't stand the thought of not being able to raise them, of leaving just an imprint where I was once real. I wasn't afraid of another woman raising them; in fact, I thought many times about wanting them to feel the love of a nurturing woman after I left them. What I hated was that I, their mother, would be gone.

I learned a valuable lesson from Josh and Alex—something that is so obvious it is sometimes overlooked. They taught me the true meaning of unconditional love.

When I was first told that something was wrong with me, a burning feeling took residence in my stomach. Then, the night before I found out that I had a tumor, I stood in the doorway to their bedrooms. They slept so peacefully. The weight of what was happening felt tremendous. I didn't know what illness I had, but knowing it was there was enough. They were so young and innocent, much like I had been at that age. I was afraid to leave their rooms, unsure if I'd ever be able to see them like that again.

After we found out about the tumor, I pretended that everything and everyone would be just fine. I was a heavy-weight champ, pounding the crap out of my mental images of their sadness, each punch delivered with the intent of making the images vanish. But the images kept coming back. I would imagine their puffy faces, tears streaming down their cheeks, and finally, their confusion and blank stares as they stood by my grave.

After the first unsuccessful surgery in August 1996, radiation gave me a dose of reality. I am not sure why I thought I could hide what was happening, but I wanted to try. I needed to be whole for my kids. It was the hardest thing to sit in the hospital waiting room with other patients like me. I could feel the desperation and hope to which we all clung. We were mothers, daughters, and sisters and had lives we needed to finish. Exhausted after each treatment, I'd rush home to the ones who needed me the most and I would try to give them what they needed. But after the third week of radiation, I couldn't hide the weakness in my body. My limbs were thin and atrophied; I could manage to go up the steps only once a day and with help. My physical appearance began to change. In addition to losing twenty pounds, my hair was thinning and my face was getting puffier from the steroids. Whether I liked it or not, I was relegated to the couch in the family room on the main level of our four-level townhouse. Life was going to happen around me and at times without me. My two sons, who were then three and nine, were around me and the illness the most. My stepson Cary, also nine, was going between our house and his mother's house. Fortunately, he, unlike my sons, had a healthy mom to go home to. We hired a nanny and— just like that—I became an observer in my own life. I felt like I was dangling from a cliff, safe if only for a moment. My death grip on the cliff gave me hope. And then, quickly and abruptly, the surface to which I was clinging was gone. Had I let go? Or did the surface disappear? It is a question I still think about. For me, the day I couldn't *mother* anymore became my worst day.

I realize now that that was *my* thought: I felt incapable, so therefore I became lost. But what my kids saw was their mother, alive and fighting. They were scared of the unknown, but even on the couch, or even in a hospital bed, I was still their mom. I learned from them that it was okay to love them the best way I could. When I was in the rehabilitation center, the hospital decided to put me in its new marketing brochure. It was a huge joke that even in sickness I was still working it as a model. I was photographed in a wheelchair with Alex sitting proudly on my lap.

In the spring of 1997, I shaved my head and wore a wig home. I had a baseball hat on over the wig. I remember so clearly sitting on Josh's bed with both boys beside me. I was so nervous. I looked my sweet boys in the eyes and said, "You know, Mommy's hair has been falling out, so I decided to get a haircut and wear this until my hair grows back."

They touched the wig, and then looked at me, confused. I said, "You don't like it?"

They said, "It's weird."

So I took off the $2,000 wig, allowing my shaved head to be exposed for the first time, and tossed the wig in the air. After that day, we kept the wig in the hall closet, sometimes bringing it out and chasing each other around the house with it. My favorite picture is of Josh and Alex, each kissing me on a cheek. My face is full; my hair is all gone but for a whisper of black; and we are all smiling. Pure love!

Once we moved back to Maryland, after I was told I had only one to three months to live, the boys knew things were worse. I was hardly mobile; I lay in Bob's old bedroom, in bed, high on morphine, visiting with friends who brought food and smiles. I later learned these same friends would go downstairs and cry in the hall bathroom. Life was slowly being sucked out of me. But I still couldn't bear to accept that I was dying. When we found a second chance in Dr. Epstein, the heaviness in our life started to lift ever so cautiously.

During the summer of 1997, when I was in the hospital, we were filled with hope and promises, both of which had been missing for the past year. For the first time, I felt that I could say, "Mommy will be here."

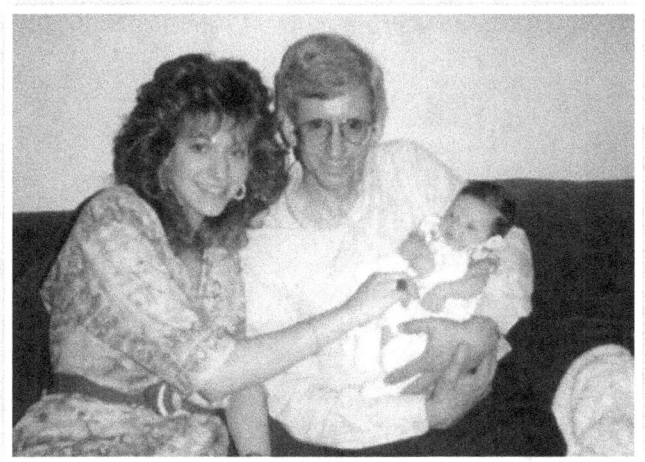

Dad and me at Josh's bris in 1987.

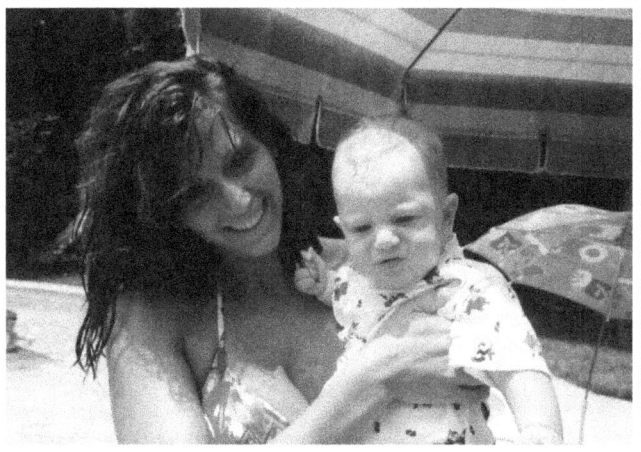

Alex and me at the pool, 1993.

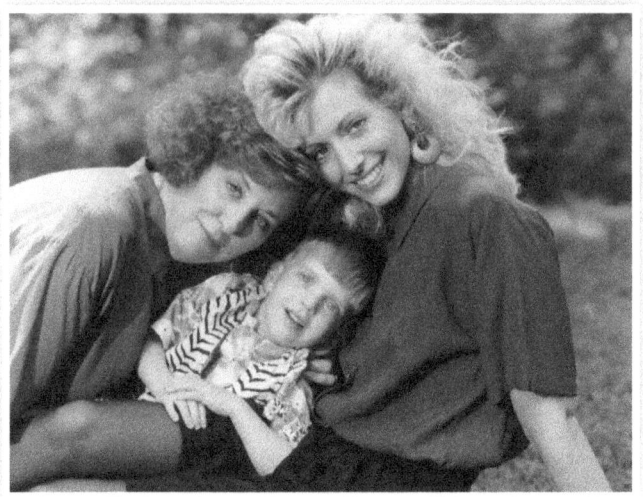

My mom, Josh, and me in 1989 when Josh was two and I was twenty-three.

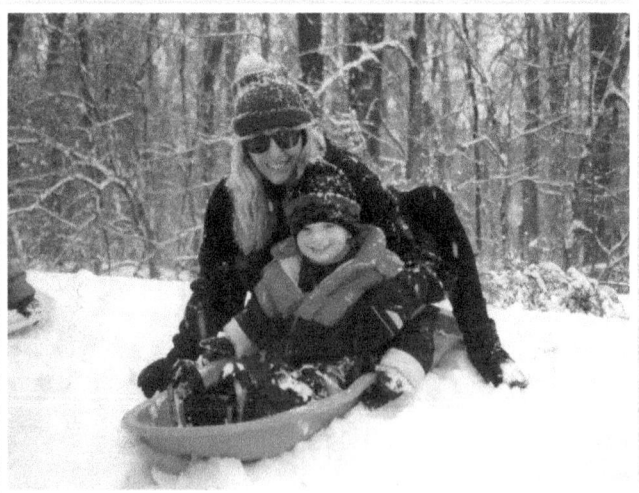

Alex and me sledding in 1995, one year before I got sick.

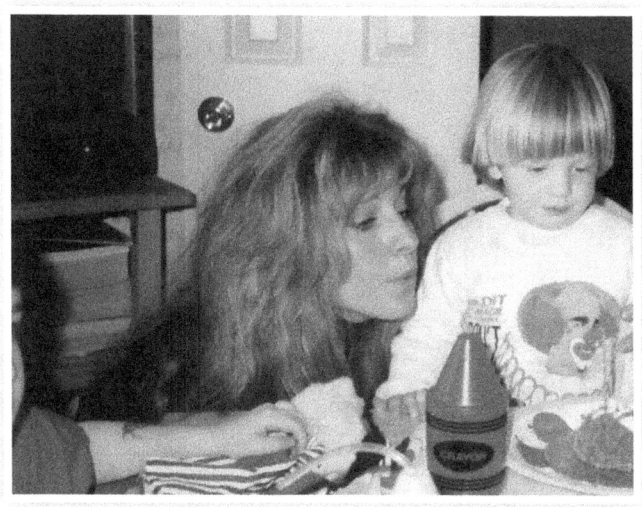

Alex's third birthday in February 1996, six months before I got sick.

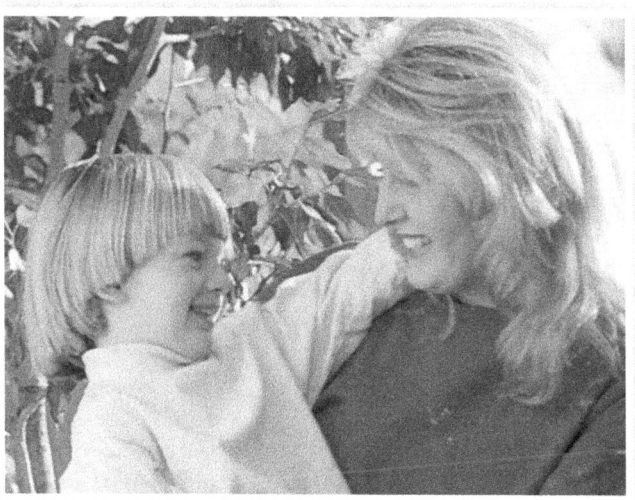

Alex and me at Bryn Mawr Rehab in November 1996. I was not walking, but we made it into the brochure!

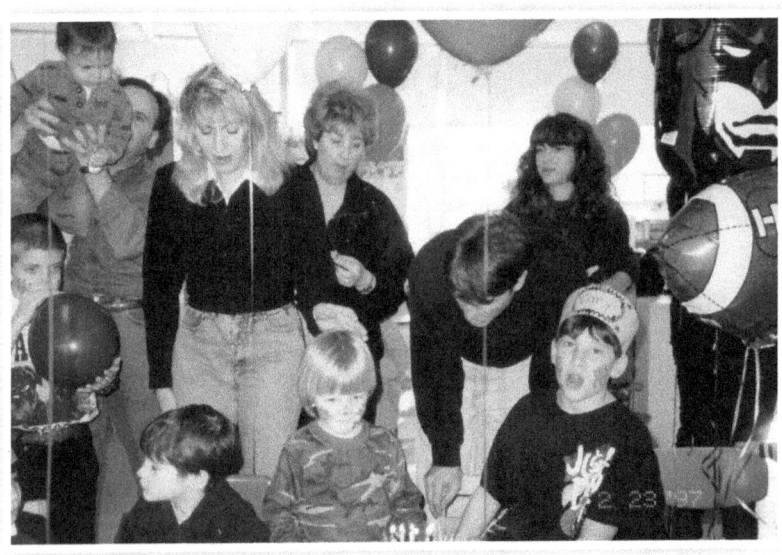

Alex's fourth birthday in February 1997. I was trying to stay off steroids.

Recovery took some time, but my boys went through it with me. Sometimes they even accompanied me to physical therapy. There were certain things I could not do after my recovery. As they grew up, I was the mom who could not go on rides because I couldn't risk whiplash. But they didn't seem to mind. We all adapted pretty easily to what I could and couldn't do. I never regained full use of my right hand, so the boys came up with an affectionate nickname: "the claw." From time to time I'd test the hand by trying to hold something, and when I dropped it, they'd laugh and say, "Was that the claw?" They are acutely aware of my follow-up MRI schedule, and they wait along with me for the results.

Throughout the past sixteen years, I have always been a little bit overprotective of my kids—okay, a lot overprotective. I know that holding onto them means that I am alive. Their young eyes saw way too much, and I wondered how my illness would impact them as they grew up. I would be lying if I said we all just moved past this horrible time and skipped our way merrily into the future. That was not our reality. Anxiety reared its ugly head in Alex years later, when he was ten years old. Josh also went to a therapist for a bit, but he definitely kept more emotions inside. He was diagnosed with colitis, and then Crohn's disease, when he was twelve, and although I know it is a medical condition with hereditary links, stress can aggravate the disease.

When Josh was thirteen and weeks away from his Bar Mitzvah and his face was swollen from the steroid treatment, I was able to look at him and remind him of how my face and body swelled when I was sick and remind him that he too would not be puffy forever.

Alex's anxiety was a different animal. Alex didn't want to be away from me or his father. I had to make him believe that he could go to school, do activities that all kids his age do, and that, at the end of the day, we would always be there, at home. But how could I guarantee that? During my illness I wasn't always home at the end of the day. It took several years, many hours with the right therapist, and time—time proved to be on our side, and day after day Alex got stronger and more confident that his world would not come crashing down on him.

Both Josh and Alex have always been incredibly brave and strong. I have been lucky enough to witness their bravery and strength over the years. Alex, always a strong athlete, focused on several different sports, and as he matured, so did his dedication to achievement on and off the field. Josh always had a passion for music. He excelled at piano and guitar. He is self-taught and writes beautiful songs, a few of which he wrote for me.

The memories of when they were young and maturing still fill me with emotion. Josh had to write an essay in middle school about who he admired most in his life, and he wrote about me. Then years later, unbeknownst to me at the time, Alex's college entrance essay was about the profound influence I had on how he lives his life. He wrote, "I will always be someone who will never quit and be the ROCK for others, just like my mother." The best part, of course, is that I am here to witness all of it. I would love to have given them a life without this illness, but to see in them such strength and passion is overwhelming, to say the least.

I became more patient as a mother. I realized that many of the pressures I had were self-inflicted. I now take moments to just be. It sounds funny to approach life this way, but when you have been dealt such a big blow, not much after that can ruffle your feathers.

Today, Josh is a college graduate with a degree in music and works as a manager in the restaurant industry; he still writes and plays piano and guitar. Alex is in college, where he is studying business and plays on the school's Division I football team. And, recently, after many years and miles apart, I have had the opportunity to spend some time with Cary.

I admit that I've made deals with God, so to speak. Every now and then, I would say, "If I can just stay healthy until they get through elementary school…through high school…until they've had their fill of me." Then it was college, and now it's, "Keep me healthy until we have grandkids…please, how about until I'm old enough to have lived a full life?" I think when you have been hit with a life-threatening illness, the bargaining is just a part of life.

Oh, how lucky I am to have these moments!

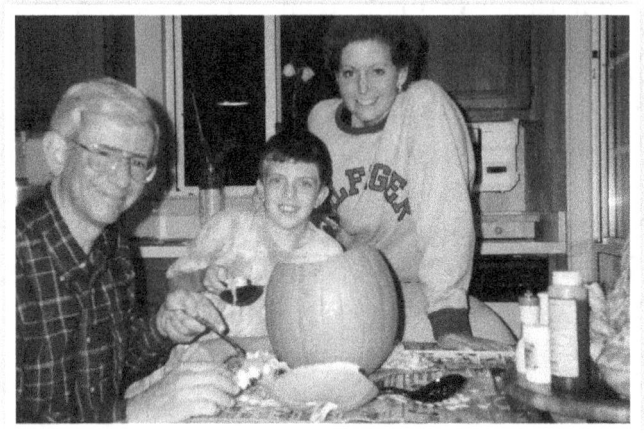

Dad, Josh, and me on Halloween 1997. My hair was growing back.

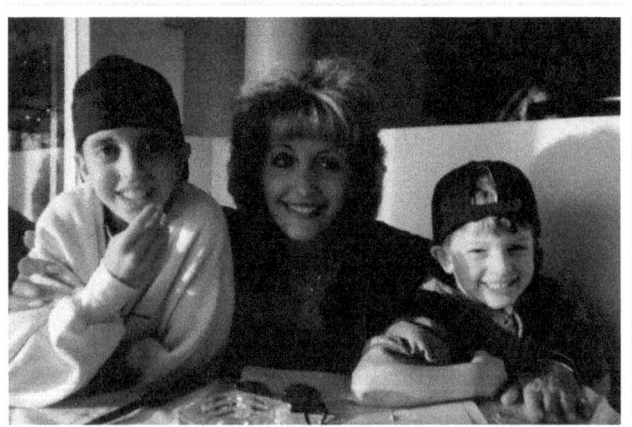

Josh, Alex, and me spending time together in January 1998.

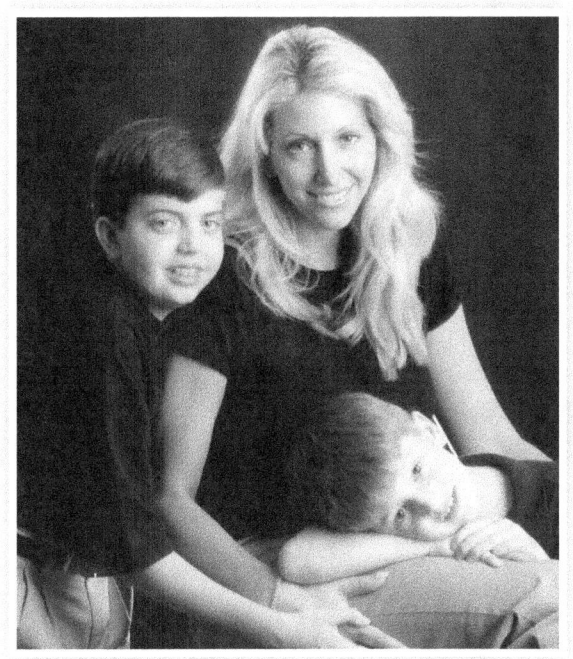

Josh's Bar Mitzvah in April 2000.

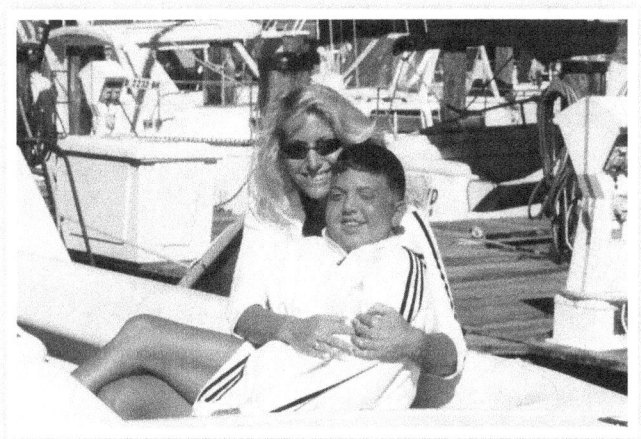

Summer 2000, Josh was on steroids for Crohn's disease.

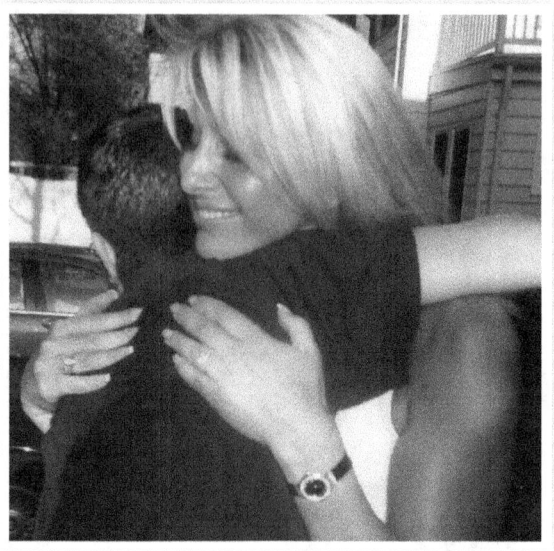

Josh gets his first car in 2004.

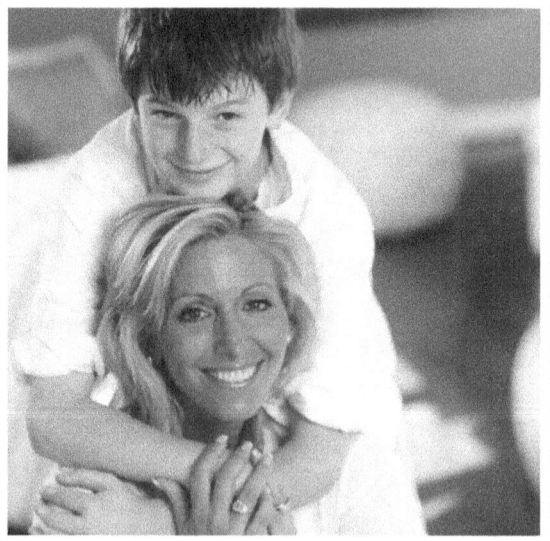

Alex and me during our casual family portrait session for his bar mitzvah.

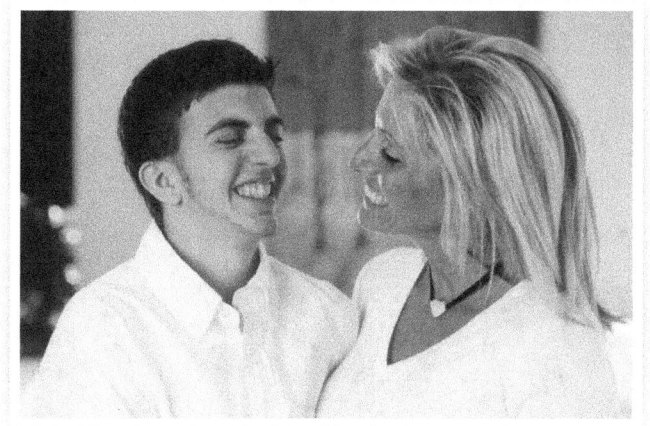

Alex's bar mitzvah in 2006.

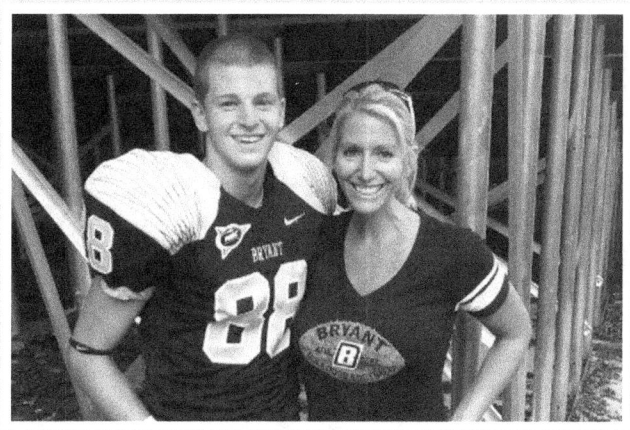

With Alex, a freshman in college, after a football game in fall 2011.

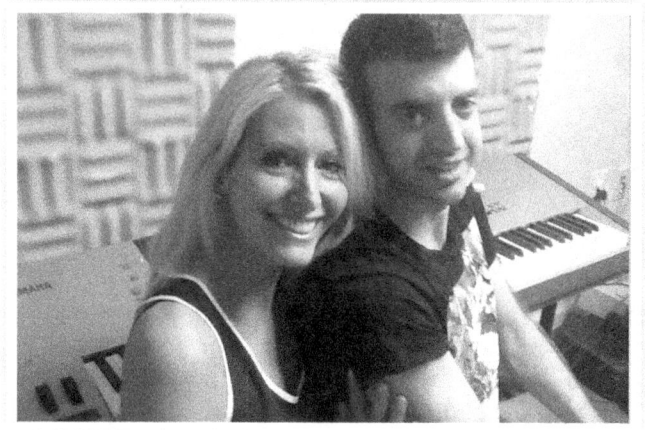

With Josh, as he records his first piano CD.

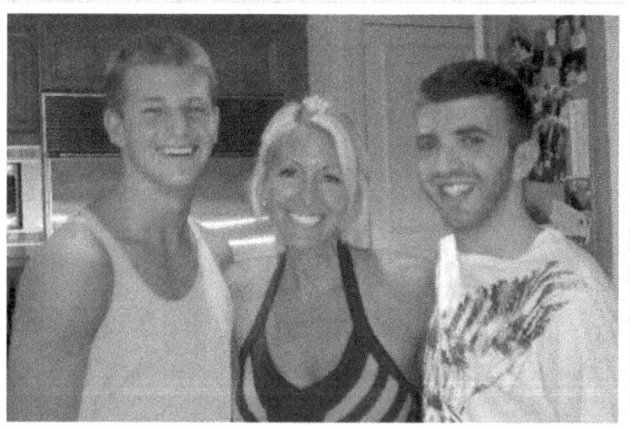

Summer 2012: one of my favorite pictures.

Reader's Thoughts:

When did parenting and being ill collide?
How did caring for your kids change?
When did you get a dose of reality?
When did you have your positive moments, who and
what gave them to you?
When did strength take over?

My Parents

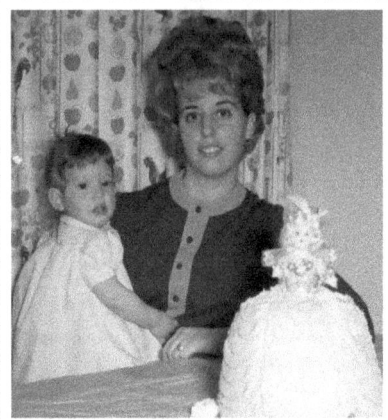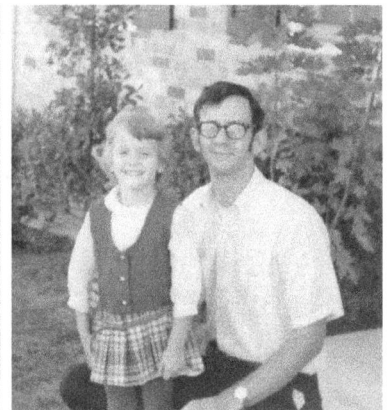

With my parents, 1966 and 1971.

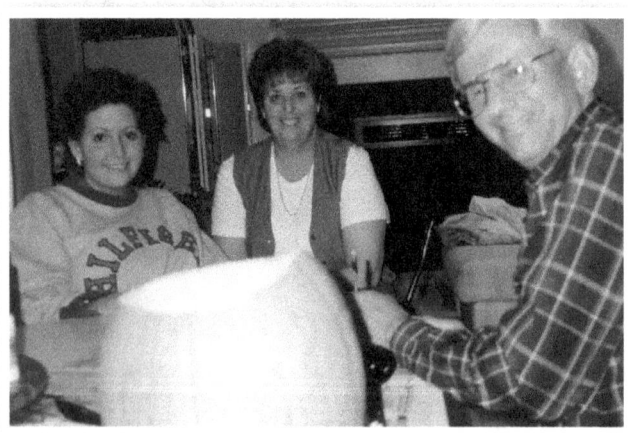

Halloween 1997

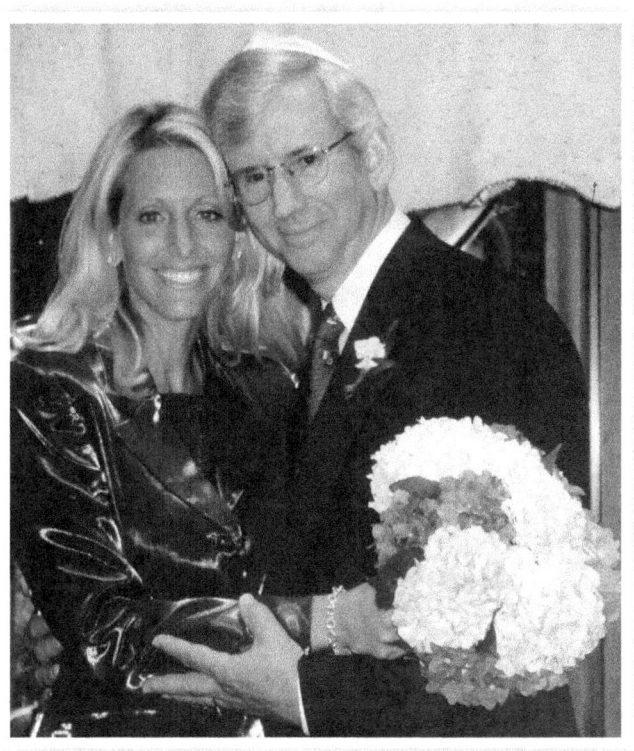

Dad and me at my wedding to Carl in 2001.

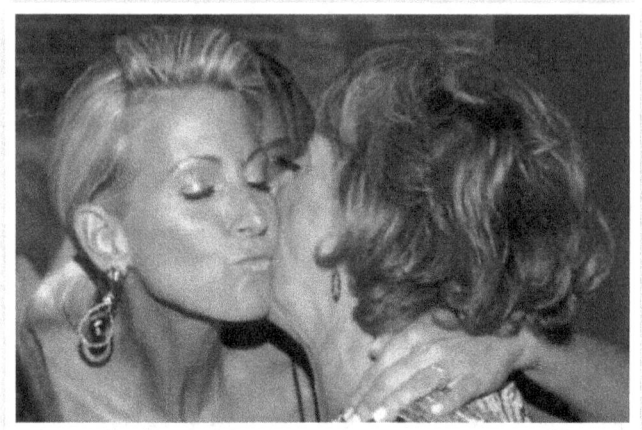

My mom…I love this picture, taken April 2011.

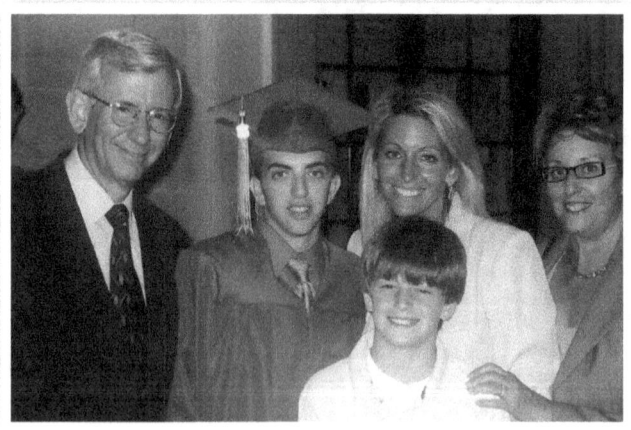

Josh's high school graduation in 2005.

3

DAUGHTER

I could not have gotten through my illness if it wasn't for my parents. My parents literally stepped up to the plate and hit a home run for me. It's important to share a conversation my dad and I had recently. I had agreed to go with my dad to a Kol Nidre service. Kol Nidre is a special Jewish religious service on the night before Yom Kippur. I say I *agreed* because, if anyone knows me, they know I am not very religious; however, I do have my own ways of honoring my faith. When I was a little girl, I would sneak into my father's car after Friday night dinners at home and surprise him when he would go to Shabbat services. So, when he asked me to go, how could I say no?

After the service that night, as we pulled up in front of my house, I told him that I was really glad that I'd gone. He stopped the car, looked at me, and said, "Me too, because sixteen years ago, I almost lost my daughter."

I have always had a great relationship with my folks. They are young and active and have always been involved in my life and my kids' lives. I am the youngest child of two and the only daughter. My brother moved away to California when he was in his early twenties, and I remain very close to him, his wife, and my niece and nephews.

During my years as a gymnast, my parents drove me to the gym every day, and for many years my gym was an hour's drive each way. They were at every gymnastics meet—just about everything I did, they were there. I was loved.

Being a sick daughter is not supposed to happen. We hear it all the time: parents are not supposed to outlive their children. It goes against the grain of life. I am lucky to have both my parents and even luckier to have a great relationship with them. When I look at my mom now, I think about the blood she gave me when I needed a transfusion—how her blood rushed through my veins, giving me warmth and life. When my kids went to Florida without me over that Christmas break in 1996, Mom came to stay with me and literally hauled my ass out of my depression. I refused to wash my thinning hair and would lie on the sofa with my lips pursed day after day, in a dark place mentally. My mom grabbed my arm and said, "Get up. Let's get in the shower. I will help you wash your hair and put on makeup. We are going out." That was it. We went to the movies.

I was using a walker, and when we got to the theater, I stumbled in the middle of the concession area and fell to the floor. I couldn't pick myself up; I didn't have the strength. She tried to help me but I was like dead weight. We both ended up on the floor. Then she stood up and, in the middle of the theater lobby, she screamed at the top of her lungs, "Can someone please help us? Can't you see my daughter has fallen?"

No one helped. My mom had to lift me herself. We cried, then laughed, and have retold that story many times.

So you probably have a good picture of my mom now: she's a tough cookie. At the time, she was running an event-planning company, the same one I would join later and eventually take over in 2011. She was nothing but exceptional and professional to her clients; it was amazing to watch her shift from her reality and theirs. But she didn't hide her fear from me. She showed it, and by doing so she helped me to realize that you *can* fight fear; it doesn't have to win.

I saw my dad cry for the first time after my first surgery. My dad is an extremely intelligent, orderly, and very loving man, a rocket scientist, of sorts. His life always had an order, a plan, and my getting sick wasn't part of that plan. I am very much like him. I like order and a plan. The difference with me now is that I leave a little breathing room. Throughout my life I called him first if I had a problem. He was my problem-solver; if something broke, he could fix it. I think that when he wasn't sure he could fix me, he himself broke, if only for a moment.

Growing up, I always heard, "I'm so proud of you." We were the family that ate dinners together six days a week at the dinner table. For as many nights as I can remember, at the dinner table he would lift my hair and gently kiss the back of my neck—a place that has a lengthy scar now that reminds us all of what we went through.

When I moved back to Maryland, after I was told that I had only a short time to live, my parents searched tirelessly to find help for me. The day we went to New York to see Dr. Epstein, I watched as my dad loaded the mattress in the back of their Jeep; then my dad helped to place me on the mattress. I remember wrapping my arms around his neck and holding on, the same way I did as a child, and the same way my own kids did to me. I felt utterly helpless but lucky to have a dad who could carry me through my most difficult time. When my parents met Dr. Epstein, there was no question in their minds that he would fix me.

My parents rented an apartment near the hospital in New York during the summer of 1997 and helped to nurture me back to life emotionally and physically. Today, we go on with our lives. My parents just recently retired and live in south Florida. I am running the event-planning company from Maryland. We remain very close. It feels like we have this extra beat that is just between us. It is hard to explain, but it is there like a smile that joins us at each turn in life. I spoke to them many times about my illness while I was writing this book. Recalling their private thoughts is still difficult. My mom's eyes grow teary and she'll say, "You know, you do what you have to do. That is just it."

Reader's Thoughts:

Who helped you break through the darkness and gain strength?

If parents played a role in your illness, or you were the parent of a sick child, what was the most difficult moment?

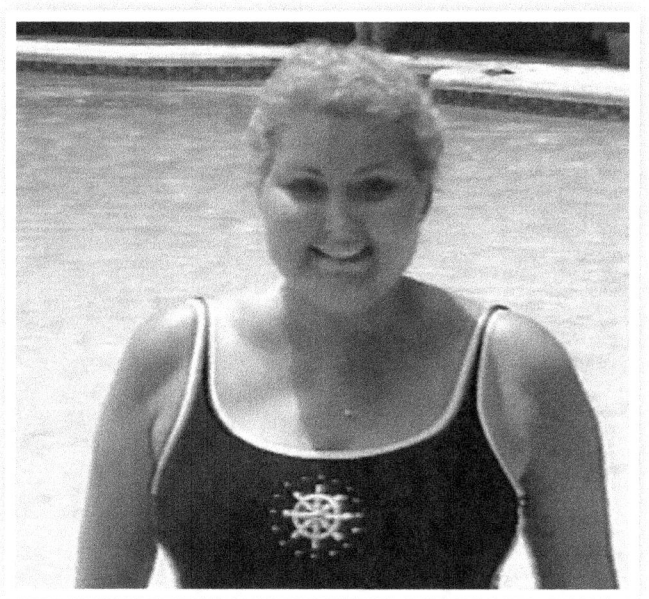

Full of hope and fear in June 1997, right before my second surgery.

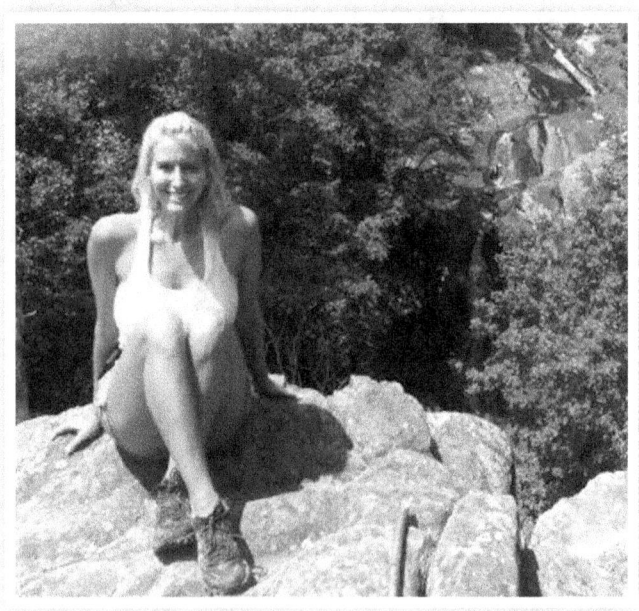

Here I am in the summer of 2012, appreciating each moment.

4

SELF-REFLECTION: "WHO AM I?"

I am intimately aware of those who cannot "look back" on their illness. The gratitude I hold in my heart is my greatest source of motivation and inspiration to see things differently, in a better light. After all, what is the purpose of going through something so traumatic if you can't learn from it and be a better person?

Not a single day goes by that I don't think about my illness. Period. The days and months that consumed me during my illness are as vivid as yesterday is. I look at the many stages that I went through much like steps in a recovery program. Of course, the steps or stages don't always progress in an upward motion, leaving you content and finally free of what ails you. Illness is a whirlwind of steps and stages. Sometimes you go up a step and then you fall back a few steps. Sometimes the ground you thought you'd gained disappears, and you have to climb back up those very same steps again.

I experienced denial, fear, anger, aggression, depression, acceptance, strength, weakness, hopelessness, hopefulness, truth, and gratefulness many times during my illness. And today, I still climb those steps.

"Who am I?" That is what I think when I look in the mirror. My whole body is a puzzle, and the pieces from sixteen years ago seem to fit in places that are visible to me at every glance physically and emotionally. Physically, I see the scar on the back of my neck, long and a little jagged, and the indentation where a bone is missing just below the nape of my neck. I see the three small, black, spots tattooed on the front of my neck so the doctors would know exactly where the beams of radiation should go. I look down to my breasts and the sides of my stomach and see the stretch marks that appeared not during my two pregnancies but when steroids made my weight skyrocket sixty pounds—twenty pounds in one month alone. I notice how my right arm hangs, not so perfectly, at my side, and I remember how I learned to become left-handed. I notice my thighs and how strong they are now, and I remember how weak they once were, unable to hold me up. I glance into my eyes, where my story plays out every day. This is who *I am*.

Today, I think a lot about what people see when they look at me. I appear healthy, attractive, fit, and, most important, happy. They assume I have no story. I don't share my story outright, so how would they know? But still, I wish they wouldn't sum me up so quickly or judge me by my cover. I have learned that by opening up a "book," you just might find a whole new perspective. I view each person I meet like this; maybe he or she has a similar story, one that's not worn on a sleeve, one that hurts to recount, and one that still brings tears to recall. But a story that made that person *who he is today*.

During the course of my illness, my appearance completely changed. Only a picture could tell the truth. I looked so unbelievably different that at times I wasn't sure it was me. I have to think that this change, in particular, happened for a reason. My illness was/is about so much more than what I physically looked like before my illness, during my illness, and now, but I would be neglecting a significant part of my illness and recovery if I didn't share this very personal part of it with you.

I was always considered pretty. I was not conceited; in fact, I was highly insecure, but, over time, having beauty on my side helped me to keep my insecurities at bay. Beauty was my crutch for so many years. So when it was gone, I became lost. I realize how that sounds. But for my entire life I had been sized up by my looks. When my life was spiraling out of control from my illness, I became confused about how I got to look the way I did. I learned that medicines and bad side effects were all to blame. I had to accept that I couldn't control what was happening. Accepting how I looked became a new challenge, and those "illness" steps came in and helped me learn how to live with this other me.

This outward change took some time for all of us to adjust to. After all, I didn't wake up one day and look different; it happened over a period of about six months. My kids would refer to me as "new mommy." Friends who I hadn't seen in a while would do a double take, stare into my eyes, and then show recognition. I also had the rare opportunity to see how strangers reacted to someone who doesn't fit into the "norm." What is "normal" anyway? I can't lie: it was hard. And I had to build up the confidence to carry this new me around.

Funny story: when I met with Dr. Epstein right before my surgery, Bob held up my modeling contact sheet and proclaimed, "This is what she used to look like!" Nice, right? But in reality, we were all shocked that I didn't look like Debbie anymore. Dr. Epstein, ever so keenly aware of how deeply this change had affected my husband, said, "Don't worry. We'll get her back to that." The day of my surgery, Dr. Epstein pinned up my photos in the operating room.

I made a video for my family about a week before my final surgery. I put on a one-piece bathing suit and stood in the pool in my in-laws' backyard. I was sixty pounds heavier than normal, my torso swelled like a prize bull's. My face was the roundest and fullest it had ever been and my hair looked like a Jew 'fro dyed yellow. My idea for the video was that the beginning would be a photo montage of sorts depicting the history of "us" my husband Bob and the kids, the end would be me talking to "them" from the pool. I spoke about this last-ditch surgery and how I hoped it would all go well. I smiled big for the camera. Today when I freeze that frame, I see me. I see the hope in my face and the fear hiding behind eyes, but most importantly I see how beautiful I really was.

There is no doubt in my mind that my mental health was at its weakest and darkest when I was sick. Today I use the experience to be more patient, compassionate, and strong every day.

I met someone a while back. He is an ER doctor and shared with me his latest book about being just that. I in turn told him about this book. I e-mailed him a few chapters and he wrote back, "Now tell me what you were most afraid of." Of course, I assumed maybe he hadn't read what I had sent. It was clear to me that my emotions were written down, but when I reread what I'd sent, I agreed that I had only scratched the surface. It was hard enough just to write down what was on the surface; I wasn't sure I could go deeper because then I would have to feel the pain again—pain I wasn't sure I could handle.

When I looked back at my previous writings, I realized this was consistent with most essays I had written. I realized that there was an "acceptable" level I would go down to, a level where I felt safe, so to speak. But I now knew that I needed to really dig into the wound. By doing that, writing became more therapeutic than I ever thought it could be. Dying is a fact of life, and realistically I know that it is impossible to have control over when and how that happens. But—and here is my big *but*—I never thought I'd die young. But who does? It is the ultimate betrayal in life; it's unfair and it is tragic. I had made a life for myself. I had children who I would have the privilege to nurture for life, right? Wrong! So how do I move on from such a close brush with, well, not existing anymore?

My answer was: I just have to. What choice did I have but to build on my experiences? I want to share just a few stories that embody my experience then and now.

* * *

What Does *Will* Have to Do with It?

There are many ways that *will* can come in and go out of your life. When I entered the rehabilitation center in Malvern in the late fall of 1996, I was in my darkest place emotionally and physically. I was severely depressed. I was on so much medication that one day I was screaming that I was pregnant, even though I had my period; another day I thought I was levitating, and on another day I actually had perfect vision, even though I am near-sighted. All of these bizarre occurrences were caused by mixtures of and withdrawals from my medications. Physically, I had lost the ability to walk on my own and use my right hand. I had no *will* when I entered Bryn Mawr Rehabilitation Hospital. And I wanted everyone to know it. The doctors and nurses, day after day, would ask me to please try during physical therapy. Some days I would just lie on the mat, refusing to go any further. I felt that this had to be hell. I would look at the other patients, mostly people with head-trauma injuries, diabetic patients who had lost limbs, and stroke patients. No one seemed to be happy or better; we all seemed to be working toward adapting to our new situations. And that is what I didn't understand. I thought that my physical condition was temporary (denial) and that I would not have any lasting effects. During occupational therapy, the nurse would show me how to carry a coffee pot to the stove and then to the table. I would ask why; I already knew how to do that. The nurse would explain that I needed to incorporate my wheelchair or walker into my actions. I was shown how to get up off the floor if I fell, using my walker for leverage. I was shown how to get on and off a bed, in and out of the shower, all with my walker and props. None of this made sense to me. I was convinced they had the wrong patient chart. So, of course, until I accepted where I was physically, I couldn't move on.

Illness descends on you like a tidal wave. It covers everything and leaves nothing untouched. You watch it start at a certain point: maybe it seems miles away, then just beyond your reach. You know it's coming but you don't know how quickly. You try to run away from it but you can't. Then in a split second you are drowning. I felt caught underwater, unable to breathe. My will did not kick in until I accepted my new reality. But then I dug so deep that I exploded out of the gushing water. For me, acceptance felt just like that.

Once my *will* kicked in I worked hard, even joking with the therapist that she didn't have to show me how to fold a bed sheet with one hand because I had a maid at home.

I was told that when I could get to the entrance of the hospital without my wheelchair, only using my walker, I could go home and continue therapy as an outpatient. I had a goal, and, within a couple of weeks, I did just that.

Sweet Eve

During my last hospital stay at Beth Israel North in July 1997, I initially shared a room with an elderly woman named Eve. She was about eighty at the time. We had only a few days together because I was moved to Dr. Epstein's special pediatric area of the hospital, the INN on the eleventh floor. Eve had had a stroke. Her family would come to visit; I would hear them tell her to fight, that her life was not over. They kept telling Eve she would recover from her stroke. She moaned and then wept when they left. I was told by her family that she had been an avid tennis player and extremely active before the stroke. I literally could *feel* her will slipping away. I didn't know her at all, and our medical histories were so different, but I would talk to her from my bed, trying to convince her that she still had so much life ahead of her. I needed her to be strong because I was trying to be strong, too. If I was fighting, she had to fight. But in the end, Eve decided she couldn't fight, and she died in her sleep. I think about her a lot. In a few days' time, she taught me so much.

Too Young

Dr. Epstein's eleventh floor at Beth Israel North Hospital was called the INN. Patients were mostly young children and young adults. I was the senior resident. We all had a common denominator: Dr. Epstein and his brilliance. We each battled different demons: brain tumors, spinal cord tumors, malignant and nonmalignant. I met so many of these brave young warriors. And each step I took toward recovery made me want to take each of them with me. I never thought I was that bad off. How could I be when at every turn was a young child fighting for his or her life? In many physical therapy sessions, we would pass large balls to each other. Even though we were improving our mobility and working on our coordination, there was an element of play. I remember thinking that this was quite possibly the closest many of these children would ever come to playing in a schoolyard. I have to say that nothing is more sobering than to watch kids try to live. Plain and simple, they wanted to live, and so did I.

Reader's Thoughts:

How did *will* enter into the picture?
Did your appearance or a loved one's change with illness?
Who do you see in the mirror?

5

WIFE

Writing this chapter is definitely one of the most challenging tasks for me. My husband Bob and I are no longer married. We both have moved on with new loves, new spouses. Writing this book the way I wanted to, I could not possibly omit something that was so central to my life. And that was being married at the time of my illness. Bob and I had been married for four years when we found out about my illness. From the moment we found out about the tumor, we shelved any marital issues. It was as simple and decisive as that. It is in both of our natures to take care of something, to make someone better; so Bob did what comes most naturally to him. He dove in. We were fortunate enough that he worked for his father and therefore could take off from work—as much time as he needed.

Bob did all he could, physically and emotionally. He fed my insatiable appetite on many occasions and sat with me during far too many doctors' appointments. He carried with him the weight of our world. He also had to deal with family, friends, and, most importantly, our children. He gave hospital beds and rehab rooms an overhaul so they would feel more like home. Family pictures and special blankets were always part of any room I inhabited. Whether out of love or duty or both, it doesn't matter. I don't think people can say how they would handle being the caretaker of a sick spouse until they experience it firsthand. It wasn't always pretty and we were not always polite to each other. I hated feeling like I couldn't be a wife in every sense of what a wife is. But like every other role my illness affected, I had to take where I was at that moment and find a way to live through it better.

There were, of course, some uniquely funny times as well, like when Bob brought a bagful of unpaid bills and the checkbook to the hospital. I was always the one who paid the bills and even though I couldn't use my right hand and was on morphine, he was determined to have me "pay the bills!" His family was large and always there for me, for us. They were a crew that rallied. When *tumult* (Yiddish for "shit"—at least that's my translation!) hit, they ate and ate more and laughed. Our marriage did eventually end in January 2000. Bob will always be the father to my son, Alex, and the person who most intimately took care of me at a time when just living was in jeopardy. When we said I do, it was for better or worse. And of course on the day of my wedding to Bob, I never imagined that there would be anything so horrible in our lifetime together. And even though our marriage ended, when the worst hit, we went through it together.

Reader's Thoughts:

How has illness affected your relationships?

6

NEW LOVE...NEW LEASE ON LIFE

Luckily, I got another chance at love. My husband of eleven years and counting came into my life in the spring of 2000, not long after Bob and I separated, and at a time when my own health and future were still unknown. It was only a few months after I met Carl that I had to go back up to New York for my yearly checkup with Dr. Epstein. After my second surgery in 1997, I went to New York for checkups every six months, and then eventually, once a year. As unexpected as love is, so was Carl and how open he was to going through what may lie ahead for my kids and me. I remember thinking, "Is this guy crazy?" In reality, that trip to New York was probably the single moment I can think back to when I knew this guy was a keeper.

It was so strange to take this new guy on a trip to see my doctor—and not just any doctor but Dr. Epstein. I wasn't sure how this whole appointment would turn out. How could I assure Carl that I was actually going to be all right? Would

Dr. Epstein answer all his questions? Was Carl going to have questions? I was definitely stressed but at the same time excited that Carl would meet the man who saved my life.

I knew I had to allow as much openness and honesty as possible during my appointment; after all, I needed Carl to be clear about what was going on with me. As soon as we entered Beth Israel North, I gave Carl the five-cent tour of the famed eleventh floor, otherwise known as the INN. Then, as we were walking down the hall toward Dr. Epstein's office, Dr. Epstein appeared, walking toward us. He stretched his arms out to me and said, "Ahh, there's my miracle." I melted in Dr. Epstein's arms, looked at Carl, and knew this was so right. Then of course I had to explain who Carl was.

We spent the next hour or so talking about my life, my MRI, the symptoms I was having, and what was next. It was a very reassuring appointment for both of us. The truth was, and still is, that because 10 percent of the tumor was left in my spinal cord, I have to continue to get MRIs. Now I have them every two years. There is a 25 percent chance that the remaining piece could start to grow again or that another tumor could branch off into another area in my body, or that whiplash or a neck or spinal cord injury could cause paralysis or worse. But isn't life filled with what-ifs and maybes? Carl and I left the appointment feeling uplifted. I think he felt some kind of relief at knowing the facts.

When I was at Beth Israel North in the summer of 1997, my hospital room overlooked Gracie Park. Every day I would look out the window and wish that I could simply stroll through the park. And on more days than not, I wondered if I would ever be able to walk again without assistance. So on that day, after we saw Dr. Epstein, Carl and I did just that. We walked around Gracie Park. I cried, and we laughed, and that moment we shared is seared into my heart and soul.

Carl didn't disappear after that appointment; in fact he dug his heels in and never looked back. We married in 2001, and I gained another son, Austin, now thirty. Carl has been an amazing husband and, most importantly to me, unbelievably kind, loving, and nurturing to both Josh and Alex. It was not an easy situation. Talk about having emotional baggage— I have a life-threatening tumor! But as he will always remind me, "I have a lot invested in you; I know what I signed up for!"

We have had a few scares since we have been together. In 2004, while celebrating a friend's birthday, Carl was accidentally pushed on top of me while I sat in a baby pool filled with Jell-O (yes, Jell-O). The fall caused my neck to crank to one side and crack. I thought I was paralyzed. Needless to say, the party ended, the ambulance came, the entire hospital staff thought I was covered in blood, and then when the ER found out it was red Jell-O—well, you can only imagine. We were terrified that I couldn't move. The prognosis was that my spinal cord had received a shock. I had a spinal cord sprain and a stinger, like what a football player gets when his arm goes limp, but I would not be paralyzed, thank God! It took about a month to recover and be able to get back to *my* normal. After consulting with my very good friend, Dr. Wayne Olin, who is one of the nation's top neuroradiologist, I followed up with a local neurosurgeon in Maryland (see next chapter about the new doctor). Dr. Aulesi, my new doctor, then lectured me about what I really can do and what I should not be doing. Jell-O pits definitely fit into the "what not to do" column.

Of course, we have retold the Jell-O story dozens of times, but the reality is, at that moment, when I couldn't move, we both thought the worst had happened, and when I looked into Carl's eyes, all I saw was fear, not regret.

We have had many blessings over the past eleven years. One of my fondest is walking down the aisle at my stepson Austin's wedding to Jamie in April 2011 with Josh and Alex at my side. Each new day brings new adventures. Sometimes life moves so fast, but I never forget where I came from.

Photos

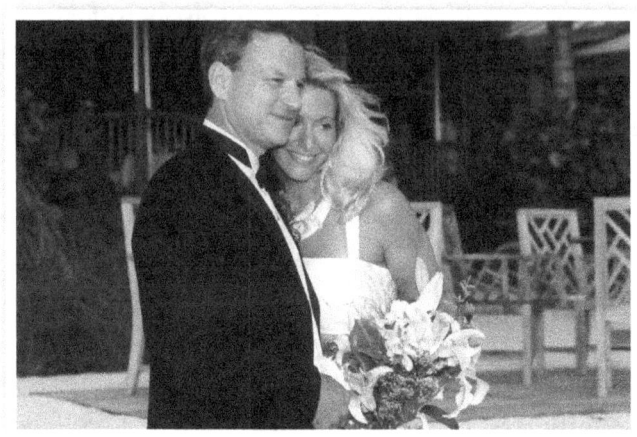

Carl and me on our "beach" wedding day, April 2001.

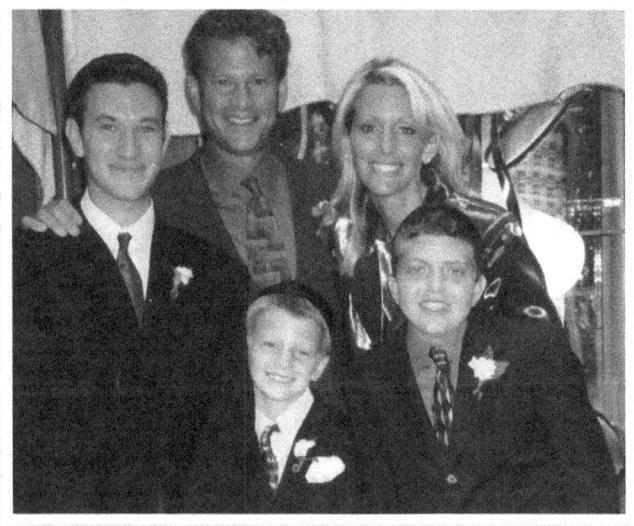

Our religious wedding ceremony 2001 with the boys.

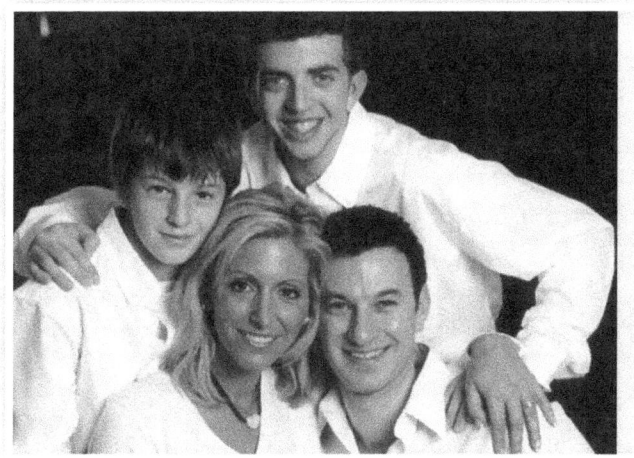

My boys and me: Austin, Josh, and Alex in 2006.

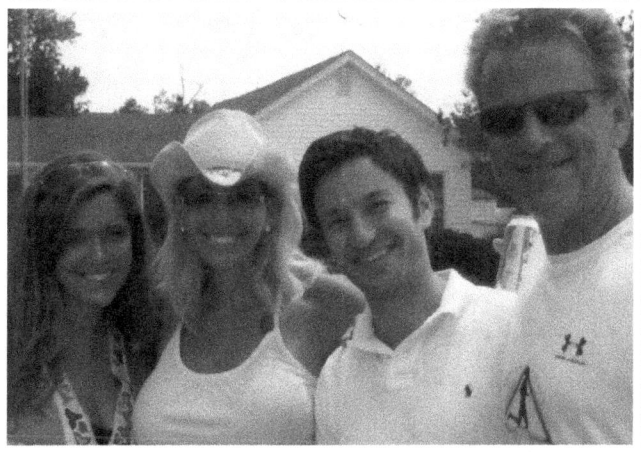

My beautiful daughter-in-law, Jamie, with Carl, Austin
and me in summer 2010.

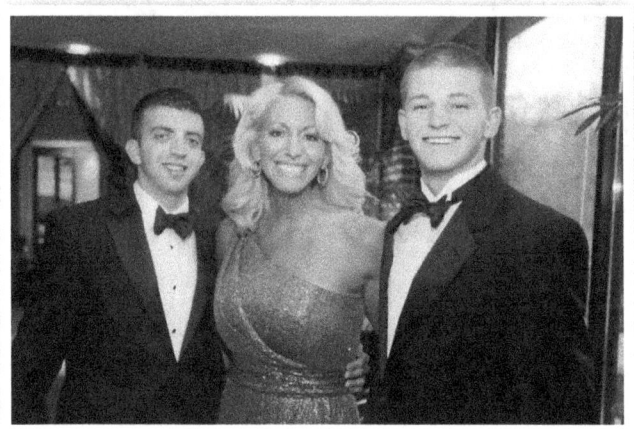

At Austin and Jamie's wedding in 2011. I was thankful to
have both Alex and Josh walk me down the aisle.

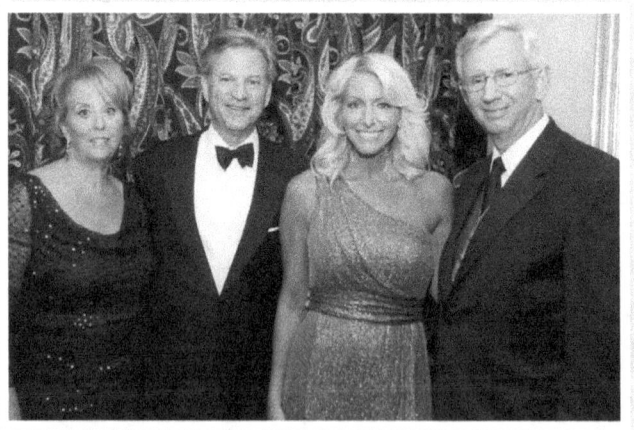

Austin and Jamie's wedding in 2011.
Photo credit: Clay Blackmore

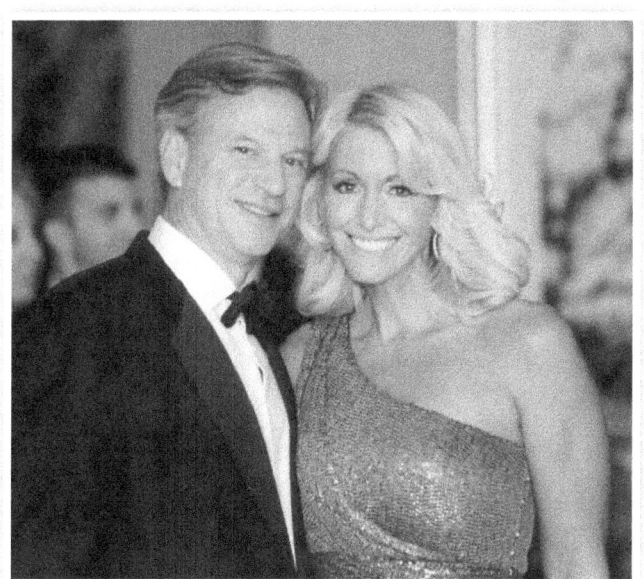

Carl and me, 2011.

Reader's Thoughts:

Did a new relationship happen during or after an illness?
Are you overly cautious about new relationships?

7

DR. FRED EPSTEIN

This man was God to me. I say that so often when I'm retelling my story. I only wish that he was still here today. I know there are many people who feel the same way. I was so lucky to have found him. From the moment I met him to the last time I would ever see him, I knew this man would always be part of me. I sometimes pull out his books and flip to the back cover, just so I can see his face. He was larger than life, but, when I was with him, in his office or in the hospital, he made me feel like I was his only patient. I read his books, which made me love him even more and allowed me to see a man, not just a doctor. He was rare and honest, and he saved me.

In 2001, four years after he operated on me, Dr. Epstein had a horrific bicycle accident that caused brain damage and some paralysis. In 2002, his wife Kathy sent a letter to all of his patients. Her letter told about the accident and requested that people share their stories of survival. "What helped you get through the worst part of your personal crisis?" she asked.

Dr. Epstein was writing a book with the help of his wife and his colleagues. In her letter, his wife expressed that they didn't want patients to write about how great a doctor he is but rather about themselves and their own personal journeys. That is just the kind of man he was. It took me a long time to come to terms with why such a brilliant man, with years of wisdom to share, could meet this kind of fate. About a year after I received the letter, we were sent an invitation to attend his book signing in New York. My mom and I went. I had no idea what to expect. The room was filled to capacity with children whose lives he had saved, their grateful parents, and with the presence of those whom he could not save. I knew from reading his books and getting to know him that each child who didn't make it still resided in his heart and soul. I was not prepared to see him in a wheelchair, but when he spoke with the help of his wife, I saw him, right there in front of me, no less than the man he was before. He was just as large a presence as he ever was. I was one of only a few adult patients there that day, which made me even more grateful. The emotions flowing were so tremendous.

I was reluctant to find a new doctor, in part because I was afraid to let go of him. I knew I would never find another Dr. Epstein. I did find a wonderful neurosurgeon in Maryland, Dr. Edward Aulesi, and the first time I went to see him, I told him who my previous doctor was. He paused and then gave me a smile that assured me he knew exactly where I was coming from.

In 2006, I got a second letter from Mrs. Epstein, only this time the letter told of Dr. Fred Epstein's death from melanoma. I was inconsolable. I began to research his death online and found an incredibly well-written article about Dr. Epstein in the sports section of a New York newspaper.

I wrote the author about my illness and my own experiences with Dr. Epstein. It was therapeutic to write to someone who seemed to have known him. What I didn't expect was to get a response back. Not only did the writer know him, but she was a patient of his as a young teenager in the summer of 1997. We were in the hospital at the same time.

Fred Epstein touched so many lives, and, because of him, so many lives prospered—not only his patients' but the professionals he taught and who now implement what they learned, in turn saving more lives. This was to be his legacy. I still wrestle with his untimely accident and death, but I know how lucky so many of us are for the time we had with him.

A percentage of the proceeds from this book will be donated to the Fred J. Epstein Pediatric Care Foundation.

Reader's Thoughts:

Who were your medical heroes?

8

FRIEND

look at friendships as the glue that keeps us bound to each other, unlike blood or duty, just by making the choice to be in someone's life. I couldn't imagine writing this book without sharing how great many of my friends were during my illness as well as the finer points of what it means to be a friend and when it's okay to receive help. Some of my friends from that time are not in my life anymore; there were some whom I needed to purge from my life and a few who just drifted away. Many are lifelong friends because when things got really bad, they hung in there with me. That is a loyalty like nothing else.

I have always been the good listener, the shoulder to cry on, and the friend who carries the weight of the world at any given time for a friend. I am a giver but I am not as comfortable receiving. That changed when I got sick. I didn't have to ask for help; my friends were just ready to serve. It was hard for me in the beginning; I didn't like to feel needy. But slowly I began to understand that helping me helped them. They needed to be part of my illness and be there for whatever might come. It was a way to cope.

I have just a few "childhood" friends, and one of them is Helene. We have been friends for forty years. (Just writing that number scares me!) She now lives in California. We have gone through every part of each other's lives together. Marriages, children, illness—you name it. I truly believe we are soul mates. The night before my first surgery in Philly, in August 1996, my husband, parents, siblings, and I stayed at a hotel near the hospital. I remember speaking to Helene on the phone before I went to bed; she lived in Maryland at the time. When I woke up from surgery she was next to my hospital bed. I thought I was dreaming, but I realized I wasn't. She was crying and shaking her head. When she'd heard that the surgery was not going well, she had dropped everything and came to me, just like that. I was so grateful. She gave me a different source of strength that can only come from a friend.

When we moved to Philly, I left many good friends back in Maryland. Several would make the trip to visit, which I loved; they would take me shopping, to my radiation appointments, or just to the park, where we could talk. I was also fortunate to develop new friendships with women from my neighborhood, from my synagogue, and through the kids' schools. These women rallied around me during my illness and were a great support system. At the end of my radiation treatment, in an effort to lift my spirits, we had an end-of-radiation party. We placed my "hockey mask" on a pedestal and danced around it like some weird tribal group. But in all seriousness, these friends cooked for my family, drove my kids to their activities, and at times drove me to appointments. The time they gave to my family was priceless.

On one of those days, my friend Amy, whom I met in our neighborhood in Malvern, took me to the mall. I wasn't able to drive at the time, so she drove. This was during my radiation treatment, and I wasn't feeling well at all. I had been taking a slew of vitamins, which, mixed with all my other medications, produced a stomachache so severe that I wasn't sure I'd make it to the restroom. I told Amy I was going to find a bathroom in the mall and left her in one of the stores. Unfortunately, I didn't quite make it, and by the time I got to the restroom stall, I needed a change of clothes. I didn't have a cell phone, and I couldn't put my clothes back on. So I was naked in the stall, alone. I remained in the bathroom stall for two more hours. It seemed unlikely that no one would help, but that is exactly what happened. It was not a busy restroom. I had used up all the toilet paper, and at one point I covered myself with the toilet lid liners so I could wash myself at the sink and then retreat back into the stall. I broke down a few times, scared and wondering how the hell I was going to get out of the bathroom. A few people came in during those two hours, and when I asked for help they ignored me. Finally someone who worked in the mall did help. I gave her money to buy me sweatpants and a T-shirt and to call my friend, Amy, to come pick me up. The funny part is that for some reason, Amy thought because I was feeling sick I had decided to call Bob and go home. She, of course, felt awful. Now it's a story that makes me laugh—I mean, really, naked in a stall with no way out... think of the one-man show that could have been! Several years later, after my recovery, Amy's mother passed away. I stayed by her side for an entire week and did everything I could to help. It was a small way to thank her for all she did for me.

I have many new friends now who didn't know me during my illness but learned about it through my stories. They have supported me by checking in after a doctor's appointment and being good listeners when I talked to them incessantly about this book. And they can't wait to throw a book-signing party! Friends even helped me train for and complete a half marathon, a 13.1-mile race, which my friend, Lisa, and I both knew was so much more than a race for me. The reality is, at this point in our lives, we all have stories to tell and pain that lives within us. Knowing you have the support of friends makes living through it easier. Having my friends see me when I was ill and vulnerable was raw and at times embarrassing. But they did not shy away, and that was and is truly a blessing.

Reader's Thoughts:

Who were the friends that stayed with you?
How have your friendships changed?

9

GETTING TO HERE

I have struggled with writing my story for many years. I wondered what place my story would have. Who would really care about one person who struggled with a deadly noncancerous tumor? What makes my story so different? Sure, my illness single-handedly defined my life, but is my story really readable? And there was my answer. Yes, it is, because just like I want to meet and talk to people who knew Dr. Epstein, I want to help people who have suffered or are suffering.

Every time I tell my story, people are moved. There are millions of people who tragically lose their lives every day. I survived. We need each other. We need to share our stories so that we can move forward.

I finally started to write my story three years ago. I had been working on a fiction project with a wonderful writing coach, Marilyn Horowitz. When I decided to shift to a memoir, she said that sometimes it takes fifteen or more years to write about something so traumatic. I guess she was right. I have consulted several people during my writing process, among them Paul Bodner, my favorite (and only) uncle who has always been a confidante of sorts for me. He is always supportive of me when I take on my next adventure. When it was acting, he sent me a book aptly titled *The Casting Couch*. He is a writer, and a successful one, at that. Whenever we would visit each other, we were consumed by conversation about our projects, so much so that my mother and aunt would just say, "We'll see you both in a few hours."

Last February he came to town and I met him for dinner. In no time we were talking about our current writing projects. As always, the conversation was intoxicating. Not only did he listen intently, he understood me. He retitled my book, suggesting that my working title was a little depressing and that "POV" gave a greater meaning to my story.

He totally got it. He understood that I was writing this book to help others. He told me about a friend who just had been diagnosed with breast cancer, saying she was exactly who I was writing this book for. I told him that I get stuck sometimes or feel like I need a break because it is so emotional to recount everything. He said, "What are you waiting for? It's not that hard. Just write."

Just a few weeks after our wonderful evening together, my uncle was suddenly diagnosed with stage-four non smokers lung cancer. I was blown away and for a few days, somewhat numb. Then I woke up and said, "Debbie, what *are* you waiting for?" I felt like I needed to finish this for him; he became my audience.

And even as he prepared to fight for his life, he still found a way to encourage me and stay interested. He asked me to send him new chapters. I did, of course, hoping that he could connect with my words and that they would help him. My uncle has been a warrior, to say the least. He has taken cancer and put a positive spin on it in a way only he can do. His trademark humor and wit is expressed daily on CaringBridge.org for all to experience. Thank you, Uncle Paul. As you always say, "Enjoy the day and fill it with love, laughter, and lots of lemonade!"

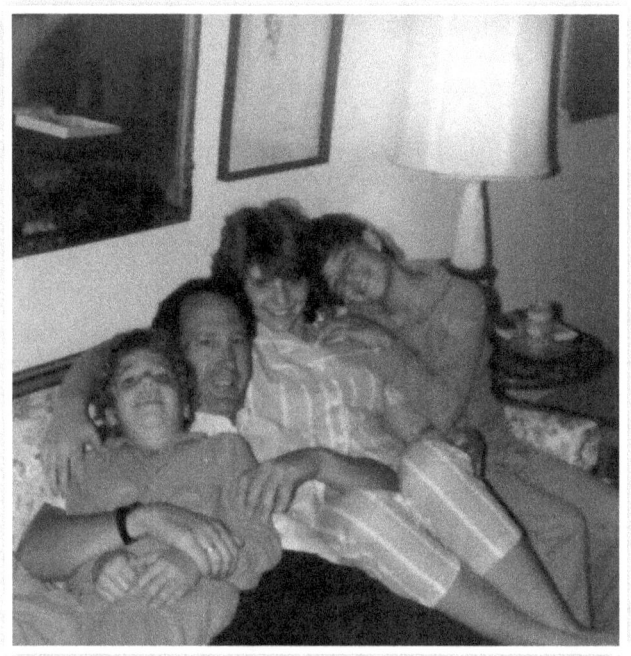

Uncle Paul, my cousins, Zack and Gabe and me in 1979.

10

SELF-ADVOCACY

can't begin to stress how important it is to be your own advocate, and when you can't, make sure your family steps in. Ask questions, keep notes, get copies, and take your time. I learned early on that just because a doctor is the head of a department doesn't mean he or she is the best doctor for you. That is the key. Ask who is the best for *me?* Who has the most experience handling my type of illness or problem?

Earlier, I mentioned seeing doctors at Johns Hopkins—who wouldn't go to Hopkins? It is a world-renowned medical center. But by researching and asking who might be better, I found Dr. Epstein. When you are ill, you are vulnerable. But vulnerability does not take away your right to ask questions and to know as much as possible about your care and course of treatment. Be as "present" as you can.

The people on my first medical team were superstars in their field, but within months, I became gravely ill from side effects; they just weren't watching me closely enough. I'll never forget telling a neuro-oncologist (even though my tumor was noncancerous, she was on my team because the treatment was thought to be the same) how thirsty I was during my radiation treatments. She told me to stick out my tongue and say "Ah." I did, and she said, "You are addicted to water." That was her answer. No blood tests or urine tests were done. But what was really going on was that I was becoming diabetic because of the steroids.

After I fired that team, I decided on a good but less well-known doctor in Paoli, Pennsylvania. I hoped things would be better. He, too, was an oncologist and also suggested treatments that paralleled those for cancerous tumors. Then, on that fateful day in June 1997, just months after I started seeing him, he told me I should wrap my life up because I had one to three months to live. As I look back now, I can appreciate that he said and did everything within his capabilities. But after my second surgery, I was so high on life that I needed an "I-told-you-so" moment. So when I found myself back in Malvern, where Amy's mom was dying in the very hospital where that doctor worked, I couldn't help myself. I had him paged. When he walked up to me, he didn't recognize me. I just stared back and said, "Not bad for dead." I felt better.

Of course, insurance plays a role in any situation like this. I don't want to discuss the politics of insurance, but when I had a choice to have my first surgery in Washington, DC, or Philadelphia, I chose Philly because that hospital was in the insurance company's network. Many of my choices were weighed against my insurance options. In reality, very few people have the money to support out-of-network medical costs. It wasn't until I was desperate did I throw caution to the wind and go out of network. What choice did I really have? The result: I was saddled with some seriously large medical bills, but with the financial help of my parents and my Uncle Paul, who was in the hospital business back then, I was able to pay down my debt. I was lucky.

Now, sixteen years later, insurance works differently in some cases. But be aware of your options and be your own advocate, always.

EPILOGUE

WHAT'S NEXT?

I have spent a lot of time staring at the title of this chapter. What's next? Luckily, the words suggest that there is actually something that will follow. So many people have bucket lists—lists of things they want to do before they "kick the bucket." When I think about my own bucket list, I have to be realistic about what I can do as opposed to what I want to do. That is all part of accepting where I am today. I know I won't be bungee jumping or jumping out of a perfectly good airplane. But even though I do have physical limitations, that doesn't mean that my list can't be all it can be. Setting goals and then reaching them is the sweetest form of a thank-you I can have. Writing this book was on my list, as is another half marathon in honor of my uncle. I don't know if my body will allow the strain, but I will try. And if I have to walk, well, that is okay, too.

While I was finishing this book, I found out that Austin and Jamie are expecting a baby and I will soon be a grandmother. I guess my bargaining is working. I used to think that I would have trouble holding a baby because of my right arm; well, now it's time to put that fear away. Just recently while on vacation, we had an opportunity to learn how to kite board. As much as I wanted to try it, I knew that because I can't hold on and feel my grip with my right hand, not only would it be impossible but potentially dangerous. Realizing I have limitations is hard. I have been practicing Vinyasa yoga for over a year now. At first I put my ego ahead of my body; after all, I was a gymnast—headstands and handstands are second nature to me. Then I fell on my head. Not so smart. Eventually, I realized I can still enjoy all the benefits of a yoga practice without going upside down.

Now that I'm forty-six, "what's next?" is an exciting proposition. A few years ago I dove back into acting, so I'll see where that leads me. So far I've had roles in commercials and a couple of quick background spots on prime-time shows (and by "quick," I mean two seconds!) I get nervous that a part I'm booked for will require a working right hand. So far I've managed to be left-hand dominant. But it is a reality nonetheless.

I have thought about going back to school, training to teach yoga, finishing my fiction novel, trying a triathlon... who knows what other crazy ideas will enter my head? The point is, "what's next?" is endless, and while my tumor could show up again and my body could progressively get worse from the side effects of the radiation, I can't live with "what if's." My approach to life is: *I will.*

Now tell me, what's next for you?

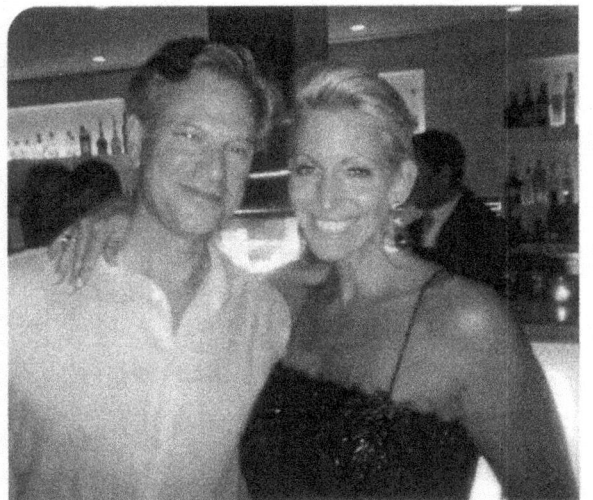

may your

HEART AND
SPIRIT
SPARKLE
AND **SHINE**

NEW
YEAR

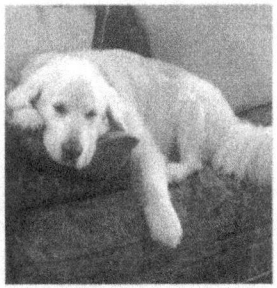
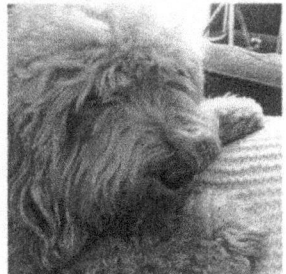
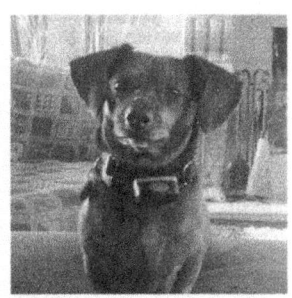

2012

warmest
WISHES

With love,
carl, debbie, austin, jamie, josh,
alex, romeo, sebi and sebastian

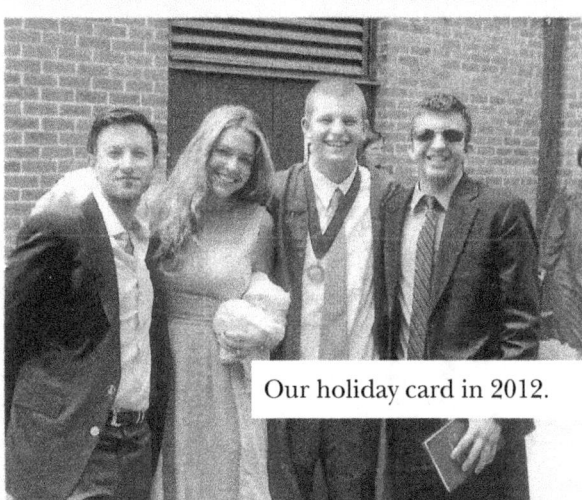

Our holiday card in 2012.

THANK YOU

This illness may have inhabited my body, but I certainly did not go it alone. Every single person who entered my life before, during, and after my illness has had a profound impact on me and my story.

Dr. Fred Epstein, you will always be in my heart and soul.

I am grateful to the many kind souls at every hospital I entered, some of whom I only knew briefly, like the nurse who bandaged Alex's stuffed monkey and tucked it next to me while I was in the hospital in November 1996. Every gesture and every kind moment has stayed with me.

Many friends have helped me with every step of this book by listening, reading, and giving much needed advice and support—Rachel, Tom, Erica R., Erica G., Helene, Jill, Jessica, Lisa N., Ross, Louis, Audrey, Lisa K and so many other wonderful friends, you know who you are. I thank each person who helped me edit, edit, and edit some more.

To Amy, Carroll, my weekly writing partner and friend, I love our writing time together. We give each other what we need and want to do: write on a consistent basis. Thank you for designing my cover! You rock! Good luck on everything you write, Amy. I already know you will be a bestseller!

To Bob, Cary, and the "Family" you were with us in the thick of it all, and your support carried us.

I am grateful to Jack Hartzman for taking my "now" photo, and the Washington Talent Team for helping me with scanning dozens of pictures, and offering your help with compassion. Davide Depas, thank you for the photo you gave me many years ago. That special image of the boys and me speaks volumes. To this day, it still gives me the chills. Marilyn Horowitz, you helped me start my engines with this book, and guided me as a writer in so many ways. I'll always be thankful for that!

To my parents, Sue and Bernie. I am just so lucky to have you as my mom and dad.

To my husband, Carl: You came onto the scene at a crazy time. Lucky for me, you were into crazy!

To Josh and Alex, you will always be my heroes. Josh, I cherish our special time together hiking and talking about this book, our goals, and life in general. Alex, your love and strength has always kept me going. I want you to always keep going strong, too!

Austin and Jamie, I am so excited to be part of your lives. I care so very much for you both.

Uncle Paul, you are an extraordinary person and full of life. I know you will beat cancer!

Thank you, to **you**, for sharing my story and yours.